D0886673

THE FRENCH RIVIERA
BODY BOOK

THE FRENCH RIVIERA
BODY BOOK

by Stephanie Sorine
with photographs by
Daniel S. Sorine

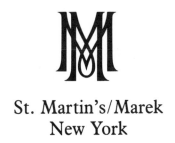

St. Martin's/Marek
New York

Acknowledgments

My deepest appreciation goes to my editor, Joyce Engelson, for her extraordinary enthusiasm and guidance, and to Richard Marek, my publisher, a great "Thank you." Special thanks are also due Joyce's assistant, Jeff Pettus, and to everyone in the design and production departments at St. Martin's Press.

Kisses and hugs to my agent, Carol Masius.

Finally, I'd like to express my gratitude and best wishes to my students—especially my mother—and to all the other people in America and Europe who gave me their time to be interviewed for this book.

THE FRENCH RIVIERA BODY BOOK. Copyright © 1983 by Stephanie Riva Sorine. Photographs copyright © 1983 by Daniel S. Sorine. All rights reserved. Printed in the United States of America. No part of this book may be used or reproduced in any manner whatsoever without written permission except in the case of brief quotations embodied in critical articles or reviews. For information, address St. Martin's/Marek, 175 Fifth Avenue, New York, N.Y. 10010.

Design by GRAEFIX

Library of Congress Cataloging in Publication Data

Sorine, Stephanie Riva.
    The French Riviera body book.
    Includes index.
    1. Exercise. 2. Physical fitness. I. Title.
RA781.S627 1983   646.7′5   82-16932
ISBN 0-312-30527-3

First Edition
10 9 8 7 6 5 4 3 2 1

IN MEMORIAM

In memory of Her Serene Highness Princess Grace of Monaco who, several months before her untimely passing, offered her time and consideration in reading this book. She generously gave it her endorsement, and we were grateful to have had the opportunity to express to her how deeply honored we were and how glad to be able to share her enthusiasm for our book with our readers.

The late Princess Grace of Monaco was devoted to the arts, health, and fitness. On her behalf we and our publisher are establishing a small fund from the proceeds of this book to be given to the Académie de Danse Classique Princesse Grace, the school she developed and loved so much.

Stephanie Sorine
Daniel S. Sorine

To my beloved husband, Daniel S. Sorine, whose love, friendship, care, understanding, encouragement, and typing skills—as well as his photographic work— helped me with this book.

Contents

Chapter 1 1
Introduction: Who Is Stephanie Sorine?

Chapter 2 5
The French Riviera Body Program

Chapter 3 9
Achieving and Maintaining
the French Riviera Body

Chapter 4 13
Getting the Most out of this Book

Chapter 5 21
Answers to Questions

**Illustrating the Benefits of the French
Riviera Body Program** 27

Chapter 6 29
The *Wind-up* and the *Wind-down*

Chapter 7 35
The 5•Minute, 7•Day Exercise Sessions

Chapter 8 109
The St. Tropez Body Plan

Chapter 9 111
More Answers to Questions

**Your Personal Exercise Chart: To Help You
Follow the French Riviera Body Program**. . . 118

Chapter 1

INTRODUCTION:
WHO IS STEPHANIE SORINE?

I'm sure you have lots of questions: Who is Stephanie Sorine? What is the French Riviera Body? What is the French Riviera Body *Program*? How does it work? Will it work for me? Well, sit back and relax because here we go!

I'm Stephanie Sorine. I've been a ballet and exercise teacher for years. Before that, I was a ballet dancer. I trained at The School of American Ballet in New York City and at The Royal Ballet School in London, England; I apprenticed with the Harkness Ballet and danced as a soloist with the Austrian Ballet. Then I had an injury, a foot injury. I was told by doctors in America and Europe that—yes—I could dance but—no—not on my toes, even if I had an operation. When you start dancing, as I did, at the age of three and a half, eating, sleeping, and breathing ballet and all that it means, *especially* dancing on your toes in pointe shoes, then it's very difficult to change your perception of yourself as a dancer. For me, at that time, not being able to dance on my toes was the same as not being able to dance, period. So that was that. In June 1975, at the Stadttheater Klagenfurt in Austria, I danced for the last time.

I came back home to America and started teaching exercise to adults and children. (Later I would teach ballet and write books about dance with my husband, photographer Daniel S. Sorine.) At first, I taught exercise programs at several establishments in New York City and in Beverly Hills, where I was on staff at Richard Simmons's Anatomy Asylum.

But it wasn't long before I felt the need to develop my own style of exercising, my own method of teaching. One of the reasons was selfish: I grew up practicing dance combinations—connecting various steps in a variety of ways—to strengthen, stretch, and increase the endurance of my body while refining its appearance and shape. I just had to find a replacement activity to keep the new me—non-dancer, exercise teacher, wife, photographer's assistant, and author—in the kind of shape I knew was possible. But I needed a method that was interesting, effective, challenging, safe, and fun. I had stopped dancing but that didn't mean I was ready to say good-bye to my size-5 clothes or the feeling of being fit and graceful. I had to create exercises that would help me, and my students.

Applying my knowledge of dancing, stretching, calisthenics, yoga, isometrics, aerobics, and anatomy, I composed what I call fitness-packed exercises—exercises that activate and benefit many areas of the body simultaneously, the way dancing does. You can mold your body into its best shape quickly, enjoyably, and with lasting effect while achieving total body fitness: flexibility, strength, and stamina plus coordination, grace, speed, control, and balance. The exercises work! Look at me and read the comments of my students in another chapter.

Having ballet in my blood has always made me strive to improve myself and perfect what I'm doing. I believe that exercising can inspire people to live a more satisfying life. That's what took me to the French Riviera in 1979 and several times thereafter.

Why the French Riviera? It's important to tell you that Daniel S. Sorine was raised on the French Riviera in Monaco among international stars of stage and screen, artists, aristocrats, European nobility and royalty, fashion trend setters, VIPs . . . and all that's elegant, sophisticated, successful, chic, glamorous . . . and, more often than not, trim, slim, and shapely. *Naturellement*, through the years Daniel had talked about the French

Riviera: the partying and the nightclubbing; the gambling in the casinos till the early morning hours; the ultra-chic boutiques; the majestic palm-tree–lined promenades such as the Promenade des Anglais in Nice and Boulevard de la Croisette in Cannes; the splendid villas; the museums; the picturesque yacht-filled ports; the sunning, swimming, boating, and tennis; the colorful restaurants and charming bistros; the ancient villages; the luxurious hotels such as the Negresco in Nice and the Hotel de Paris and L'Hotel Hermitage in Monte Carlo; the azure Mediterranean sea; the fruit and flower markets; the romantic drives; the beautiful beaches; the dazzling views of the coastline; the pleasant climate; the handsome men; the sexy women.

And knowing that I'm body conscious, Daniel frequently mentioned that the majority of people visiting or living along the French Riviera somehow always seemed to be in better shape than people elsewhere. There he rarely saw anyone in flabby condition, no matter how old or young, how rich or poor.

Of course, I was more than eager to explore what the French call the *Côte d'Azur*. I had lived in Europe for three years, traveling as a dancer through many countries, but I'd never been to this plush and spectacular international playground. In April 1979, Daniel and I hopped on an Air France flight for the first of my many visits to such resorts and cities as Monte-Carlo, Cannes, Nice, Antibes, St. Tropez, Menton, Villefranche-sur-Mer, Eze-sur-Mer, Cap d'Ail, St. Jean-Cap-Ferrat, Beaulieu-sur-Mer, St. Paul de Vence, Cagnes-sur-Mer, St. Raphaël, Ste. Maxime, Juan-les-Pins, Roquebrune-Cap-Martin, and La Turbie. It was very impressive and somewhat baffling to me to see such a plethora of beautiful bodies despite the delicious food and wine so temptingly available.

Not only did most people there seem to be in fabulous shape and condition but they also projected wonderful dispositions: parking attendants and princesses; shopkeepers and kings; waitresses, airline stewardesses, movie stars, students, and VIPs alike. No matter what their financial or social status, or where they were seen—at the beach, at work, at home, at a party, at the theater—they looked glamorous, sexy, confident, youthful, sleek, chic, healthy, energetic, and relaxed. In fact, they exuded the vitality and tranquility of vacationers, even if they weren't.

I was surprised. How did they achieve and what did they do to keep what I then named, with considerable respect and admiration, the French Riviera Body? That's what I wanted to know when I interviewed the owners of these bodies! Through my conversations, observations, and experiences there, I did discover how the French Riviera lifestyle and philosophy lead to the attainment and maintenance of the French Riviera Body itself. I found that those with a French Riviera Body:

• Realize that taking care of their bodies "is a lifetime activity for a lifetime of good living."
• Don't exercise compulsively; they're not fanatics. They may drive fast, but when it comes to eating and exercising they are sensible and do both in moderation.
• Don't necessarily belong to a health club, jogging group, or exercise class. Some of them can't afford it; some just don't have the desire or time to join or attend.
• Don't diet rigidly. They don't give up their wine, cheese, and bread but they are careful to keep snacking to a minimum.
• Exercise daily; of which they all say some version of: "I have a certain way of getting in shape and keeping in shape no matter what time of year or place I go." "It's part of my life. Every morning I do it." "I make it my business to exercise for a few minutes every day: I exercise at home in the morning, at the office before lunch, at friends' homes, on business trips, and on vacations." "Exercising makes me feel good and look as if I'm ready for the French Riviera anytime. And exercising a little bit several times a day helps me to keep my body in French Riviera shape all year."

I also found that French Riviera Body people:

• Strive always to explore their own potential, to achieve more mentally and physically.
• Want to be noticed. Their bodies say, "Look at me!"
• Believe it's wiser to prevent than to heal. They avoid getting fat, flabby, and stiff by staying in shape.
• Make time for what's important: their minds, their bodies, their families and friends.
• Keep active all day working, living, and playing . . . in addition to exercising! Because many of them do not have as many conveniences and labor-saving devices as Americans do, they must exert themselves more. They do not take their cars everywhere on short trips. Instead, they walk, ride bicycles, climb the hills and stairs.

- Believe everyone's body deserves to look good.
- Treat their bodies with respect and care.
- Want to be good lovers. "Sexy comes from inside. If you are comfortable in your own skin—happy and secure about your own body's shape and condition—then it shows and people feel as good about your body as you do."
- Feel it's very important to look and feel as good as they can every day.
- Recognize the relationship between a healthy, in-shape body and a healthy, rational, clear-thinking mind. (This is not a new philosophy born out of the fitness craze. Even in the fifth century, European philosophers thought education had to be geared toward the body as well as the mind: Man should not only be cultured but handsome.)
- Take responsibility for their own shape and condition, believing that to let themselves get out of shape is an insult to nature.
- Know that if they keep active, the years won't take a heavy toll.
- Have fun, seek to have fun, and are ready to have fun at any time.
- Care about being in style and presenting a savvy, chic, tranquil, sexy, healthy, elegant, and energetic image.
- Want to be agile and attractive for a lifetime.
- Make sure their bodies are in good shape so that they can go from their business wear to swimwear to jeans to evening wear to nothing at all without looking or feeling inhibited.

My research did not end in the south of France. I traveled through other areas of France, Switzerland, and Italy interviewing and observing people and their lifestyles. Most significantly, I spoke with many Americans about exercise, including my students. I studied and analyzed other exercise programs—particularly those covered in books—and I read what doctors and scientists had to say about the subject.

When I read that statistics indicate that nine out of ten Americans who start an exercise program quit after one month, even though America leads the world in the number of doctors, hospitals, physical educators, and others involved in health care, I knew it was imperative to find out why this was so. In order to offer to people an exercise program that they could and would stay on indefinitely, I needed to know:

- why *you* hate exercise or love it
- why you do or don't exercise

- why you procrastinate when it comes to exercising
- what would help you stay on a program
- what you want to achieve with an exercise program
- how often you exercise
- why you do or don't exercise every day
- why you do or don't exercise at home, on business trips, on vacations
- what would help you exercise every day
- at what time of day you prefer to exercise
- how you want your body to be, feel, and look
- what you like and dislike about other exercise programs
- what kind of exercise program you want and need
- how exercise affects your life

I found out you needed a program you could follow daily for a lifetime, anywhere, at any time of day or any season of the year, a program that wasn't boring, tiring, confusing, intimidating, alienating, time-consuming, or overly demanding. You wanted a program that was convenient, organized, uncomplicated, motivating, effective, stimulating, economical, sensible, and always fun to follow: a program that made it easy to get in shape and stay in shape forever.

Many of my students, among them magazine and book editors, also said, "Please write down your exercises. I need something I can follow at home." "I go on a lot of business trips and I just hate getting out of shape. I'd love to be able to exercise in my hotel room." "I'm so glad you're finally doing a book. Now I can exercise with you at any time of day or anywhere I am."

My major concern was how to create an exercise program with everything you wanted and needed in it, so you could achieve and then maintain the French Riviera Body. In this complex world, you certainly didn't need another exercise program you couldn't follow or that didn't work. So I combined my fitness-packed exercises with the French Riviera Body mode of exercising—regular exercising anytime, anyplace, with anybody—to create a practical, five-minute-a-day regimen that uses every major muscle group in your body. Here is the French Riviera Body Program for your benefit and convenience—different, challenging exercises for every single day of the week—so easy that getting in shape and staying in shape is only a matter of remembering what day it is!

Chapter 2

THE FRENCH RIVIERA BODY PROGRAM

The French Riviera Body Book comprises the French Riviera Body Program of daily exercising that can be followed by all people at any level of fitness. Scientifically designed, the French Riviera Body Program will solve your exercise problems, especially how to get in shape fast and stay in shape permanently. It helps you create a new exercise lifestyle which can be practiced and enjoyed anywhere, anytime, with anybody. Through this program you will improve your body, image, and mental attitude by attacking every figure problem from the infamous pot belly to the droopy derrière, and including thick ankles, shapeless calves, sagging chin, wrinkled neck, flabby thighs, slumping chest, weak back, chubby knees, fleshy arms, round shoulders, spreading waist, and oversized hips. You will develop your strength, stamina, and flexibility as well as your coordination, balance, discipline, grace, and confidence. All these benefits can be yours for keeps by following the French Riviera Body 5-Minute, 7-Day Exercise Sessions from now on.

Moderation and consistency are the underlying principles of the French Riviera Body Program. Exercising is effective when it is done daily in a prescribed pattern, not when it is done in random bursts of enthusiasm. How long and how strenuously you exercise is not nearly as important as how regularly and exactly you follow this program. (One of the fastest ways for you to kill your motivation is to overexercise, especially the first few days you are on this program. Overexercising is painful, and could easily discourage you from continuing.)

Although following this program fifteen to twenty minutes twice a day is what I consider ideal, you'll soon discover that even a few minutes a day can mean a world of difference to you. You'll realize that no matter how long or short your periods of exercise are, each one counts when you follow this program as described. Just five minutes a day on the French Riviera Body Program can help you look and feel your best.

Flab is a result of excess weight from overeating and muscle atrophy from inactivity. Sitting for hours every day as many of us do constricts the circulation in our thighs and buttocks, causing them to be flabby, powerless and oversized; as it also enlarges our waists and weakens our chest and back muscles. The human body needs exercise. Exercising daily, as you can on this program, cures and prevents out-of-shape ailments that modern luxuries, occupations, and lifestyles can cause.

Dieting is not enough; it does not contribute to or maintain your flexibility, strength, muscle tone, and stamina. You can't get a flat and firm stomach, for example, just by losing weight. Your abdominal muscles will still be soft, sagging, or protruding. Your posture will not improve. And when your posture is neglected, your upper body slips downward, increasing the burden on your legs, spreading your waistline, and adding girth to your lower abdomen. Poor posture (slouching) can also cause deposits of fat to accumulate on your hips, buttocks, and abdomen, generating lower back pain and fatigue. To feel and look good—to be able to live, work, and play as well as you can—you must exercise.

On this program, each day and every week your whole body will be thoroughly exercised. Not one part is neglected, and the major problem areas for fat and flab are emphasized: the hips, abdomen, buttocks, waist, and thighs. You will flatten and firm your stomach and give extra support to your body—particularly your back—reducing, preventing, or eliminating lower back pain. My exercises will strengthen your abdominal, back, waist, and upper body muscles, which will improve your posture and trim the size of your waistline and abdomen.

Through the exercises, you will be breaking up fatty deposits on your hips and losing unwanted inches, and you will also become more agile and graceful as your hip joints loosen up and the muscles around your hips become stronger. If you tire quickly when walking or climbing stairs, one possible cause is weak and sagging buttocks. The firm and streamlined buttocks you will achieve as a result of exercising on the French Riviera Body Program will look more attractive, and you will have more energy. Because your legs are exercised in so many different ways, the bulges, sags, ripples, dimples, and flab will be reduced or eliminated and replaced by leanness, sleekness, and shapeliness.

Your upper body muscles in front and back are exercised to improve your posture, making it easier to sit and walk erect. And you'll look about 10 lbs thinner without even losing a pound! Your arms—the undersides, too—are exercised to firm and strengthen them. Your ankles, toes, hands, and feet are exercised for greater flexibility and endurance. You will also learn how to release tension and stress while toning muscles in your neck, shoulders, and even underneath your chin by following the French Riviera Body Program.

This program will convince you that exercising is a necessity but that it is also something to look forward to every day. The French Riviera Body 5-Minute, 7-Day Exercise Sessions provide a concentrated, comprehensive, and unique body-conditioning treatment for you to follow each day of the week—Monday through Sunday—composed of my carefully devised and arranged fitness-packed exercises. For your benefit, both physically and mentally, each session is distinct from the others; however, all seven sessions are equally efficient and effective, because I planned all of them with the same purposes:

● To produce the French Riviera Body by activating each and every part of your body in a variety of ways;

● To be followed and completed within five minutes, encouraging you to exercise more than once a day;
● To extend and reinforce the benefits of preceding sessions and prepare you for succeeding sessions;
● To be merged with other sessions on the more advanced St. Tropez Body Plan.

Each session is individually complete, having its own set of exercises with its own internal rhythm and pattern. Monday's session begins standing, Tuesday's sitting . . . no two sessions are alike. From start to finish, each day's session is uniquely its own. This kind of variety invigorates both your mind and your body, eliminates the possibility of boredom, and benefits your body thoroughly.

The exercises have been designed in a definite order. The sequence of exercises, like steps in a dance routine, creates sessions that are exhilarating, challenging, and fun. Each exercise flows into the next so you can exercise in a smooth, sustained way, which improves the capacity of your cardiovascular system and further develops your coordination, balance, and grace. Like dancing, exercising on the French Riviera Body Program is wonderfully good and inspiring. Each five-minute period goes by swiftly as your body is seriously strengthened, aesthetically slimmed, and gracefully stretched.

There are only ten exercises in each day's session plus wind-up exercises to warm your body up and wind-down exercises to cool your body down. So whether you're following the French Riviera Body Program or the more advanced St. Tropez Body Plan, you have few exercises to deal with each time, so it will be easy for you to become familiar with each session quickly. You can concentrate on how you are doing the exercises rather than on whether or not you can endure a lengthy and complicated workout. You know that you will be able to finish each session from wind-up to wind-down within five minutes; this boosts your confidence and motivation. You can follow this program here and there during the day, every day turning exercise into a natural way of life. Your life.

The directions to each session's exercises indicate the required number of repetitions. (A repetition is each full movement of an exercise. It includes parts A and B, and C and D when applicable.) The repetitions can be decreased if you are a beginner, have less than five minutes to exercise, or are recovering from an illness. Otherwise, the number is fixed. You should exercise at least five minutes a day. You can also exercise more intensely, or more than once a day, by repeating that day's session from wind-up to wind-down or, if you are following the St. Tropez Body Plan, by merging two consecutive days' sessions from wind-up to wind-down.

Unlike some exercise programs that instruct you to do 10 of this exercise, 25 of that one, and so one, I'm instructing you to do only one to four repetitions of each exercise so you can complete all the exercises in each day's session in the promised five minutes. There are other reasons, too, for doing fewer repetitions: "Doing each exercise 25 to 50 times consecutively is so uninspiring and terribly dull." Repeating an exercise over and over again can be boring and it can overwork muscles. That's neither necessary nor advantageous, and it's also no fun. And monotony, fatigue, and pain can be forerunners to such injuries as ligamental or tendon strains, joint pains, and muscle pulls.

Repeating each exercise so many times consecutively doesn't guarantee that the quality of performance will improve. Chances are that with each repetition, your execution of the movements will get sloppier. And on this program, *how* you do the exercises is just as important as how often you do them. It's better to repeat entire sequences of exercises that put no strain on your joints or muscles but still activate every part of your body, than to sweat and strain, for example, through 50 of the same sit-ups in a row.

While too many demands and complications discourage you from starting exercise programs at all, excessive repetitions cause you to detest them or quit. That's why so many of you don't exercise or have abandoned other exercise programs—and why, once you start this program, I'm sure you won't want to stop.

To help you start each exercise the right way, a preparatory position is given. And throughout each exercise, instructions like "pull your abdominal muscles toward your back and up toward your ribs," and "tighten your buttocks," which are sometimes given as "pull" and "tighten" as well as "pull your shoulders back and down" and "hold your chin and chest high" frequently appear. (Other important instructions are detailed in Chapter 4 under "Special Tips.") Teaching exercise classes and being an exerciser myself has taught me which corrections, instructions, and reminders need to be repeated more often than others for proper body positioning and alignment

and to help you get into shape faster and more safely. For example, by continually pulling in your abdominal muscles you are tightening and strengthening them so they become superfirm and trim and more supportive to your back. Your posture and appearance improve and lower back pain can be prevented, reduced, or eliminated. Activating the abdominal muscles also trims your waistline.

I always say "tighten your buttocks" so you will shape, strengthen, and firm them to improve your appearance and increase your energy level. By pulling your weight up off your hips and increasing the space between your hips and ribs, you can actually redistribute the weight that tends to settle on your hips, buttocks, thighs, abdomen, and waist. Of course this helps to form a smoother torso and firmer, sleeker legs. No more spare tires around your middle! No more cellulite on your thighs and buttocks! And stretching your body upward also relieves the cramped and compressed feeling in your lower back. Pulling your shoulders back and down gives your upper body a look of confidence and authority and you will revel in the strength and energy that comes with having good posture.

Other general instructions: To keep your back straight while you exercise is to strengthen it. Relaxing your neck and face allows you to channel your energy to other parts of your body where it's more beneficial.

Specific breathing instructions are incorporated into every exercise description. Inhaling brings fresh oxygen to your muscles and increases your muscular strength and firmness. Exhaling rids the system of toxic gases and relaxes your muscles so they can be pulled and stretched without strain. Since you're instructed never to hold a position longer than you're able to without holding your breath, your breathing becomes a built-in device to help you set your own pace and exercise rhythmically and smoothly.

These exercises blend some of the finest techniques of ballet, modern and jazz dance, yoga, calisthenics, stretching, isometrics, and aerobics. You will recognize the grace, poise, posture, line, and use of the rotation in the hips from ballet; the flowing, relaxing, and refreshing qualities of yoga; the isolated movements of jazz dance; the style of modern dance; the strengthening, toning, and firming methods of calisthenics and isometrics; the nonstop, sustained approach of aerobics; and the trimming and lengthening potential of stretching.

Each form of activity has something special to offer, and combined they become exercises that complement and balance each other to help you develop flexibility and to give your body a greater capacity to use its full range of movements. And they give you the strength to perform everyday tasks and movements with new ease, so you'll have less fatigue in walking, running, dancing, loving, working, climbing stairs, carrying packages, playing games like tennis, and taking care of your friends and family. These exercises also promote cardiovascular fitness for endurance and stamina. When your heart and lungs are in good, healthy condition, more oxygen can be carried to your cells.

These exercises are fitness-packed. My waist stretch, for example, will not only exercise your waist but also your abdomen, hips, shoulders, buttocks, arms, neck, and more. My sit-ups will flatten your tummy and trim your waist as well as limber up your back and hips, strengthen your heart and lungs, and firm up your arms, even thighs, buttocks, underneath your chin.

Because the exercises presented here are those that I teach my students in New York City, I asked them to comment about my exercises. A film producer said, "I feel as if all my muscles are constantly being worked." An accountant added, "I've tried everything and your exercises use the most muscles. Every part of my body gets exercised." "Your exercises are concentrated," noted a model. "I get so much out of them." From the manager of a Madison Avenue clothing boutique: "They honestly work! Your exercises are not gimmicky." "They don't get boring at all," said a writer and editor of a national magazine. "I like the variety and I feel that they work every part of my body."

I've been a dancer, then an exercise and ballet teacher for many years. First and foremost, however, I'm a human being and I share with most of you those depressing tendencies to get fat and flabby. I, too, love to eat. I, too, can be lazy. And I wish a slim, trim, and firm body was something we could slip into in the morning, but it's not. There are no short cuts to achieving the French Riviera Body. But the balance this program achieves between structure and diversity, flexibility and discipline, is what makes this exercise program one you can live with and use forever.

As you will soon discover, the ability to exercise daily, get in shape fast, and then stay in shape for a lifetime is made possible because of this program's unique format and the variety and substance of its exercises. If you follow this program exactly as described, you won't abuse your body or exhaust your mind. Instead, you will get fabulous results both physically and mentally. You will achieve and then maintain the French Riviera Body!

Now, before you start on Monday, give yourself some time to learn the principles and ideas behind this program. Read all the chapters. Take a picture of yourself for future reference. Study the French Riviera Body 5-Minute, 7-Day Exercise Sessions. Plan when, where, and with whom you will exercise. Have a medical check-up. Discuss this program with your doctor and talk with him or her about any limitations you may have. Visualize yourself exercising, attaining the French Riviera Body, and maintaining it always. Then start the French Riviera Body Program!

Chapter 3

ACHIEVING AND MAINTAINING THE FRENCH RIVIERA BODY

Like the people with the French Riviera Body, you neither want nor need to be fat, flabby, stiff, or tired; you want to have fun, feel and look good, be energetic and successful. That's why I created the French Riviera Body Program: to help you attain and maintain the French Riviera Body so you can live better, longer, and happier.

You may travel often; have children to take care of; be on a work schedule that doesn't permit you to attend exercise classes; not be able to afford the fees of a health club; be afraid to run because of rising crime, injury, barking dogs, unpleasant weather. As one of my students said, "I dislike running intensely. I think it shortens some muscles that I try to lengthen, specifically the Achilles tendon, and puts too much stress on my knees and hips. For me, running is not complete; it's aerobic—good for the heart and lungs—but it doesn't do much for the rest of my body." Maybe you're embarrassed, shy, or just don't like to exercise with others; having to go somewhere and put on an outfit could be why you don't exercise. You could be out of shape, in great shape, or in between. Perhaps you're one of millions who have never exercised before and feel sluggish, old, stiff, and uncomfortably flabby.

I asked people who've never exercised before or who have done it on an on-and-off basis through the years, "Why do you regularly brush your teeth, comb your hair, eat, and sleep?" "I have to," they said. "But why every day?" I pressed. "Isn't once or twice a week or every so often enough to prevent ailments and maintain or improve your health, appearance, and sense of well-being?" "Definitely not," was the answer they gave me. So I asked, "Why don't you stop brushing your teeth, combing your hair, eating and sleeping altogether?

Wouldn't it make your life easier?" "Hey. That's a stupid question," replied one person. "You're right," I said. Then I asked them this question as I ask you now, "So why should you procrastinate when it comes to exercising daily?"

Always remember: Health—mental and physical—is your greatest wealth. But you must invest in it every day. And it's worth investing in because looking and feeling good gives you a special independence and security so you can live life to its fullest. To exercise on the French Riviera Body Program is to make that investment in yourself and to receive more benefits—mentally and physically—than the time, energy, and effort you expend.

The French Riviera Body Program makes it easy for you. It adjusts to your schedule, needs, goals, level of fitness, and lifestyle. You can start this program as a beginner, an advanced exerciser, or at any level in between. Start any Monday of your life. Follow this program exactly as described and you *will* achieve the French Riviera Body. You can follow this program in the morning, afternoon, or evening, with your family, friends or alone, whenever and wherever you want each day. You can exercise in your living room, hotel room, at the beach under the sun, on vacation or a business trip, while watching TV or your children, listening to music or a conversation, during lunch or a coffee break. Wear anything you like: night clothes, day clothes, or nothing at all. I'm wearing unitards or leotards and tights in the photographs in this book so you can see clearly how the exercises work and how to do them. Also, I'm wearing a different kind of outfit for each session so that you can easily distinguish one session from another.

The French Riviera Body Program gives you the

freedom to exercise, to get in shape, and to stay in shape. Because it's a portable program, exercising is always possible, a convenience that makes "keeping up" easy and fun. You don't have to rely on machines or other people, or spend extra time and money to attain and maintain a sleek, fit body. You can do it yourself on the French Riviera Body Program, and I'm here to guide you.

All you have to do on this program is exercise and enjoy the results. You don't have to pick and choose exercises from all over a book, flipping pages back and forth to get some exercising done, since that difficult and tiresome process of devising and arranging exercises into distinct 5-minute, 7-day sessions has been handled for you. I know the more details you have to worry about when exercising, the less energy and time you have for the actual exercises. The whole process can become depressing and intimidating. So I worked out what you should do, in what order, on which day, so you can smoothly and naturally make exercise part of your life. The page flipping, shuffling about, and Chinese-menu types of programs ("Do two from page 3; do one from row 12 and three from row 2; repeat #6 from page 8 only twice a week . . ."), the going forward and backward and mixing and matching are too mind-boggling. I've provided you with a sustained and rhythmic exercise program that will accomplish almost everything you want.

Not only aren't there pages and pages of isolated exercises in this book from which you are expected to concoct your own program, but I also don't make further demands on you to skip rope, lift weights, run for miles, work up a sweat, feel burning pain, or dance in "The Nutcracker." It's unreasonable to think that you would or even could exercise daily if you had to deal with all that or to repeat the same old exercises each day at a specific time and for a specific amount of time unless it was convenient, practical, and enjoyable for you. And what good is an exercise program if you can't stick to it?

I don't put pressure on you to exercise for long periods of time. I believe, with scientists, doctors, and people I interviewed who have the French Riviera Body, that in exercising, frequency is more significant than intensity; regular exercising, even a little each day, is more valuable and beneficial by far than exercising sporadically—doing a lot one day and then nothing at all until days later. And it's infinitely more valuable and beneficial than not exercising at all. Sure, I understand cramming in

lots of exercise to lose those extra pounds in a hurry; or running around all weekend after sitting at a desk all week. But the big run on Saturdays, for example, does not get you into good shape. In a poll conducted by *The Los Angeles Times* in 1981, sportswriters, sportscasters, orthopedic surgeons, coaches, and professors of kinesiology were asked to rate athletes' fitness. The athletes who got the highest marks were those who had no off-seasons.

On this program, you exercise daily. You don't shock your body by movement or allow stiffness to set in. You don't start the whole process of conditioning each time you exercise. *Au contraire!* You progress quickly and retain your accomplishments for a lifetime as your body builds flexibility, stamina, and shapeliness that last.

I don't use intimidating or threatening tactics. First of all, I wouldn't like it if it were done to me; and second, I know from my own experience and from others' comments that as soon as you start doing these exercises, as soon as you see and feel how quickly and wonderfully they work, you won't want to stop doing them. Again, let me quote my students: "When I exercise regularly," remarks an actress, "I'm in a much better frame of mind. I rarely get depressed." A mother of three children told me, "When I don't exercise, I feel awkward, tired, and flabby." A salesgirl said, "When I exercise I feel so good physically, I'm happy. It helps me diet; after exercise I don't want to eat fattening things." A secretary reported, "I'm finding exercise to be fun and I look forward to it. Besides that I'm getting intrigued: I want to be able to touch my head to my knees so I have to keep doing it to see how I'm progressing." An opera singer does my exercises because: "I have to look and feel my best. Feeling in shape is part of feeling confident." "I look more radiant," says a copywriter at an advertising agency. "It's fabulous for the skin." A domestic who takes my exercise class adds, "I just love when my friends ask me what I'm doing with myself to look so in shape." And, finally, my own mother tells me, "I think that it is the best thing that could have happened to my life."

The French Riviera Body Program is addictive. You will want and need to exercise daily to circulate your blood, stretch your muscles, and feel strong, firm, trim, youthful, and more relaxed. (Researchers have discovered that exercising leads to a natural and healthy sense of well-being because it stimulates the production of substances in the body chemically similar to some tranquilizers.)

And the French Riviera Body is easy to maintain—just continue the exercises at least once a day every day—so that once you have it, you can have it forever.

There's no trick to following the French Riviera Body Program or staying on it. No complicated theories to memorize. No money to spend on special equipment, fancy exercise outfits, or running shoes. No gimmicks. No gadgets. All you have to do is follow the French Riviera Body 5-Minute, 7-Day Exercise Sessions and the wind-up and wind-down exercises exactly as described. You must! It's the best way to integrate exercise into your life and get the results you want and need. You will develop a lifetime pattern of exercising so the French Riviera Body Program and the French Riviera Body simply become a part of you. Otherwise, you'll soon slide off the program and, of course, won't get the desired results. It's fine to be casual, but to get in shape and stay in shape you have to be serious and follow the French Riviera Body Program as it's explained here: Do Monday's session on Monday; Tuesday's session on Tuesday, and so on. Or, Monday's session with Tuesday's and Tuesday's with Wednesday's . . . if you are on the St. Tropez Body Plan.

The program was constructed like this for your benefit. The body and mind respond best to exercising daily with a variety of exercises—rather than the same ones every day—and by following an organized program. By alternating the muscle groups utilized, you can lose inches, firm up, trim down, and get strong without depleting your energy or enthusiasm.

So follow this program from now on! Start on any Monday and never stop. You will never again have to say about exercising: "I don't have the time," "I'm too tired," "It's boring," "I don't have the discipline," "It's too hard," or "I hate it." Now, you won't get out of shape in the winter and go crazy getting back into shape for the lighter clothes and swimsuits of spring and summer. You don't have to gasp every time you look in a three-way mirror, or turn down dates, stay home from parties, postpone skiing week-ends or your chance to go to the French Riviera. You can get off that merry-go-round of getting into shape and out of shape, going up and down the scale and in and out of proportion. You can get and keep the French Riviera Body and be at your best, always.

Allons!

Chapter 4

GETTING THE MOST
OUT OF THIS BOOK

*T*he *French Riviera Body Book* is meant to teach you about exercise: how to do it, what it does for your body, and why you should do it. But its principal raison d'être is to provide you with a lifetime exercise program that enables you to exercise at least once each and every day.

One or more times a day you do the wind-up exercises on pages 29–33, plus that day's session, Monday through Sunday, then the wind-down exercise on pages 33–34. Or, if you're on the St. Tropez Body Plan, you do the wind-ups, that day's session, and the wind-down plus the next day's session from wind-up to wind-down.

This program is simple and it works! Once you have the sessions down pat (and they're easy to learn), all you need to remember is the day of the week! In time you can acquire the French Riviera Body through the French Riviera Body 5-Minute, 7-Day Exercise Sessions but, of course, only if you follow this program exactly as described. And here are some basic rules, special tips and extra treats to help you:

Basic Rules

1. Start this program on any Monday, any time of your life. *But first get your physician's approval.*

2. Follow this program at any time of day, wherever you are or may be going, all year round.

3. Do each session only on its appropriate day and in the sequence described. For example, when it's Monday do Monday's session. On the St. Tropez Body Plan, when it's Monday, do Monday's and Tuesday's sessions.

4. Don't skip a day unless you're ill or it's an emergency. But if you do have to skip or miss a day, don't assume that there's no point in continuing this program. Just start again with the appropriate day's session. If you are ill on Tuesday and ready to recommence on Wednesday, do Wednesday's prescribed session.

5. Do the wind-ups before you start any day's session and always finish with the wind-down exercise.

6. Don't substitute, or add or subtract repetitions, exercises, or sessions unless indicated or recommended. But if you have a special problem with an exercise, go on to the next one. Leave that exercise out of that session for a week or two and reinstate it when you feel ready for it.

7. Work into this program gradually, especially if you've never exercised before or are very much out of shape. For the first week, do each session from wind-up to wind-down only once on that day. Subtract one or two repetitions from each exercise. Omit the exercises marked with an asterisk. If necessary, modify the exercises as instructed. During the second week, do each session from wind-up

to wind-down again only once a day, but don't subtract any repetitions. The third week you are on this program, you can begin to increase the length of your exercise periods and follow this program more than once a day as described in rule #11.

8. Follow the French Riviera Body Program for at least four weeks before you go on to the more advanced St. Tropez Body Plan.

9. Try to follow this program for at least five minutes a day; your maximum exercise time is left up to you. Once you are used to the program, exercise for 5–10 minutes each day for good results; for very good results, 10–20 minutes each day; for excellent results, 20–30 minutes each day; and, for optimum results, 30–40 minutes each day.

10. Follow this program once a day or several times a day. Do one long exercise period or spread out your maximum exercise time by doing two, three or more exercise periods throughout that day.

11. In order to follow this program properly more than once a day and to increase the duration of your exercise periods, repeat *only* that day's session—or those days' sessions if you are following the St. Tropez Body Plan—from wind-up to wind-down *no matter how many times you repeat them.* For example, on Mondays, only follow the exercises associated with Monday. If you are following the St. Tropez Body Plan, follow only the exercises associated with Monday and Tuesday on Mondays, from wind-up to wind-down, of course.

12. Do the exercises without interruption. Make the transitions from part A to part B (and C to D, when applicable) smooth. Don't rest between exercises. That's how to get the most out of your five minutes.

Special Tips

General Tips

● Don't wait until you lose weight to start the French Riviera Body Program. As you follow this program and develop the exercise habit, you will realize that you burn calories more efficiently, diminishing the need to diet. You will also have more control and discipline to handle the kinds of stresses that lead to overeating, smoking, drug use, sleeplessness, depression, and related symptoms of an unhealthy lifestyle.

● If you've just had a baby, it is important to consult your physician before starting this program. Generally, one can begin this program two to four weeks after a vaginal delivery and four to six weeks after a Caesarean section.

● Before you start your exercise period, you may want to take a warm bath or shower. It's a good way to loosen up your muscles and joints.

● If you like to delay getting out of bed when you wake up, you can do many of the exercises from the wind-up chapter while you're still lying down.

● You may wear whatever you want to exercise, but it's better if it's something comfortable which allows you to move freely.

● In order to stimulate and challenge your body and mind, you should try to do each exercise at a different speed (being careful always to perform the movements as directed).

● Although you only need a small space for the sessions, it's a good idea to shift around those few furnishings which may be precariously located.

● You may want to use a towel, mat, or rug for those exercises you do lying down.

● Similarly, use a pillow or a cushion if you find leaning on your knees uncomfortable.

● Avoid drinking alcoholic beverages and eating heavy meals before exercising. If you do either, wait at least one hour before you start the session.

• Exercise in front of a mirror occasionally. As accurately as you can, try to imitate the positions and movements of my body, as they are pictured and described.

• Work hard but don't push or strain. A little huffing and puffing means you're conditioning your heart and lungs and improving their efficiency.

• Sweating is part of the body's cooling and ventilating system. You may or may not work up a sweat. It depends on your physiological make-up, what shape you're in, and how hard and long you exercise.

• Be sensible! Don't exercise to the point of exhaustion.

• Never get upset, frustrated, or discouraged about how high you can lift your leg, how far you can reach or bend, and so forth. It's a waste of time and energy. You need not have athletic abilities to follow this program or to benefit from it. Be assured that if you follow this program as specified, within a reasonably short time you'll look and feel markedly better. And, as a bonus, your legs will go higher and you'll be able to bend and reach farther for longer periods of time as your strength and flexibility increase.

• During the first week you follow this program, your muscles may feel sore as a result of being revitalized by so many fitness-packed exercises. You may experience a pulling sensation along your muscles as you stretch to increase your flexibility and body tone. Don't quit. Don't even skip a day. The fastest way to make the soreness disappear and to get your body accustomed to this program is to keep doing it. Take warm baths and showers, too. They're always soothing.

• Make a goal. What would you like to look like and how would you like to feel? Write it down. Know what you would like to accomplish, then pursue your goals. So many of my students never thought they could reshape their bodies—especially in the arm, buttock, thigh, abdomen, waist, and hip areas—and feel so good doing it.

• Once you have reached your goal, remember how you used to feel and look before you started this program and what your original reasons were for buying this book. If you want to keep the French Riviera Body and don't want to regress, you must continue to follow this program.

• Don't put this book on your bookshelf. That's not where it belongs. Let The French Riviera Body Book become part of your environment as the French Riviera Body Program becomes a natural and steady part of your life. Pack the book in your suitcase or slip it into your bag or attache case wherever you go—to friends, family, the office, on business trips, or on vacations.

• Treat this book like your toothbrush and following this program will be like brushing your teeth.

• Don't overlook any chance to follow this program: Exercise while your nails dry, when you're watching T.V., listening to music, minding the children, as you're waiting for tea, coffee or whatever to brew, during telephone conversations, or while you're waiting for a delivery or repair person to arrive.

• Wake up a little earlier to do your exercises. It will be more beneficial than the sleep you'll miss.

• Whenever you're sitting for a long period of time, take a break and follow this program. Sitting too much cramps and tires your back, widens your waist, and spreads your derrière out of proportion.

• At work, you may want to schedule your exercise periods as you would meetings, or do them whenever the opportunity arises. Wear whatever you already have on or slip into your "exercise clothes," which you can keep in your bag, desk, or locker. When you take a 5-, 10-, or 15-minute break with this program, you'll feel and look more refreshed, relaxed, and ready to tackle the rest of the day's activities.

• If you exercise before going to sleep, do it slowly to relieve tension and stress and help you become drowsy.

• For easy access when you wake up, put this book on your night table and leave it open at the wind-up chapter before you go to sleep.

• Most of us don't have the very long lunch periods they enjoy on the French Riviera, where they often take anywhere from two to four hours to eat, exercise, and chat. So make your time quality time. Simulate the restfulness and revitalization of a long and active lunch time by following this program before you eat.

• Instead of snacking, follow this program. Exercising renews your energy, boosts your spirits and makes you firmer and more flexible. Compare that with a cup of coffee and a danish or a bag of chips.

• After work, if you go directly home, follow this program. Then take a leisurely bath or an exhilarating shower depending on how your day went and how you want your evening to go.

• To reduce stiffness and fatigue while you are traveling, do the exercises in the wind-up chapter suited to your seating or standing arrangement.

• After a long trip, follow this program. Exercising feels especially good after sitting or standing still for hours.

• Fill in the chart provided in this book and write down when, where, and with whom you will exercise. Make sure you fill in the chart with schedules you can follow, then stick to your plans. But exercise whenever an opportunity arises.

• Use the "Comments" area on the chart to write down your goals, achievements, scheduling reminders, problems, changes.

• If you should want to expand your daily exercise time, but still don't have a block of time to set aside, you can spread out your exercise period into five-, ten-, and fifteen-minute segments. It's the same amount of exercising no matter how you slice it up!

• Consider scheduling shorter periods of exercise whenever you feel like skipping a day.

• Examine your Personal Exercise Chart (see p. 119) every few weeks. You can quickly see whether or not you are faithfully following this program and what you may need to do to get back on the track.

• If you seem always to be missing one particular day's session, substitute that session for another once in a while.

• If you have less than five minutes to exercise, you can still do that entire day's session from wind-up to wind-down with only one repetition of each exercise.

• If you've got the French Riviera Body but you've been ill, resume your schedule of exercising gradually. Working with your chart, make your maximum exercise times less than they had been prior to your being ill. When you have fully recuperated, return to your usual schedule.

• Make extra copies of the Personal Exercise Chart and put it on your refrigerator, in your bathroom, by your scale, in your closet, in your bag or case, on your desk, near your calendar, on bulletin boards, and wherever else you can readily see it.

• You may want to make extra copies of the chart to have available for your future use. By the time you have filled in the chart in this book, however, you should no longer need it. You will already be in the habit of exercising at least once a day.

• Get out your piggy bank. Each time you finish an exercise period, drop a coin or two into your bank. While you are benefiting physiologically and psychologically—daily, quickly, noticeably—you will also be benefiting financially. With the money you save, treat yourself to something special.

Specific Tips

Having proper body alignment and exercising with precision, balance, and control helps you to get the most out of your efforts and avoid sprains and strains. Keep these specific tips in mind as you do the exercises but don't fret if you don't get them all right at first. It will all fall into place in time.

• Don't grip the floor or the insides of your shoes with your toes. Uncurl and extend them during exercises.

• Follow the prescribed breathing instructions as you do these exercises. If you find yourself holding your breath, you've held your position too long. Move faster if you must. Controlled breathing increases your stamina and decreases stress on your heart and lungs.

• Imagine a line running the length of your foot from your second toe to the middle of your leg. Bend your knees along this line directly over the middle of your feet. Don't twist your knees by bending them inward toward your big toes.

• When you're asked to turn your legs to the outside, turn them only so much that you are still able to bend your knees directly over the middle of your feet.

• In order to stretch your Achilles tendons and tone your calves when you bend your knees, make sure you relax your ankles and toes and try not to lift your heels off the floor.

• When you flex your feet back at the ankles, it should feel as if you are pushing out through your heels.

• When you flex your hands back at the wrists, it should feel as if you are pushing out through the palms of your hands.

• When you point your feet, don't forget to point your toes.

• Don't arch your back when you pull your shoulders back and down. Keep your back straight.

• When I tell you to tighten your buttocks, you should feel the muscles contract from the outer sides of your "cheeks" to the backs of your thighs.

• When your hands are on the floor, stretch your fingers straight. Don't curl them.

• Relax your face and neck. It's easy to become tense in those areas while you're exercising.

• Stretch your knees and elbows only as much as you can. If at first you do not have enough flexibility to straighten them completely, do whatever you can. Don't give up! Flexibility comes by exercising your body, not by neglecting it.

• To prevent dizziness, stand up slowly from low positions. Put both feet on the floor. Bend your knees. Lower your head aiming your chin to your chest and slowly roll up through each vertebra to stand erect. Relax your arms. Breathe easily. Don't lift your head or straighten your knees until you've straightened your torso.

• When your legs are together, pull your inner thighs toward each other for toned and firm thighs.

• When you bend sideways, bend from your waist and keep your lower body still. Bend directly to each side without swaying or tilting your hips.

• To strengthen your back, prevent strain, and improve and correct the alignment of your spine, press the small of your back down to the floor while lying on your back or exercising on your back. It's helpful to tilt your pelvis slightly upward to the ceiling and slightly inward toward your ribs.

• Jump at an even pace and as high as you can. But, unless jumping high is important in your life, don't worry about the height—or lack of it—of your jump.

• Use your whole foot to jump up and land from a jump. When you push off, roll through your feet from the heels through the balls of your feet, pointing your toes as you leave the floor. Land by rolling through your feet from your toes to your heels.

• Straighten your knees as you jump. Don't forget to bend them as you land.

• As you land from a jump, don't cave in at the waist. Keep your back straight, your abdomen and buttocks tight, your shoulders down and back, and your chin and chest high.

Extra Treats

• Stand correctly when you're exercising and when you're not. Distribute your weight equally between both feet and on all toes. Be light on your heels. Pull your abdominal muscles in toward your back and up toward your ribs. Stretch your spine upward, increasing the space between your hips and ribs. Tighten your buttocks. Keep your shoulders back and down and your chin and chest high. Don't lean toward either side or put all your weight into one hip. That way of standing seems to cause bulges in the thighs, commonly known as saddlebags.

Learning to stand correctly whether you're exercising or not can help you eliminate now and prevent many problems in the years to come, including dowager's hump, lower backaches, and ankle and foot afflictions. Good posture also instantly improves your appearance and gives you an energetic image.

• Don't slouch or slump when you're sitting. You put a strain on your back and weaken your chest, abdominal, waist, back, and shoulder muscles. Instead, sit up straight. Pull your abdominal muscles in toward your back and up toward your ribs and stretch your spine up from your tailbone through your neck.

• Keep your abdominal muscles pulled in tight and your chin and chest high when walking.

• From time to time, shake out your hands and feet, wiggle your toes and fingers, move your shoulders and head around in a circular motion, and breathe deeply to release tension and to increase the circulation of your blood and your energy level.

• Also use everyday situations to keep active. The more active you are, the more food calories you use up and the fewer there are to settle as fat and flab on your body.

When you're doing housework, twist, turn, bend, reach; vary the speed at which you work. While you're waiting for a bus, train, taxi or your date, tighten your buttock muscles, pull in your abdominal muscles, and correct your posture. Climb stairs instead of riding escalators and elevators. Walk whenever you can—inside your house or apartment, in a park or shopping mall, on your lunch hour, after dinner, to the grocery store, to your friends or family, to the post office, to a restaurant, to work, and even when you're talking on the telephone. The brisker the better. Don't always use your car for short trips and if you have to take a bus or subway, get off a few stops before your destination and walk the rest of the way. It's much more liberating and invigorating to walk than to sit or stand in a crowded, stuffy bus or subway or to fight traffic.

• Don't always carry or hold your handbag, tote bag, shopping bag, attache case, suitcase, telephone, etc. on the same side. Your spine becomes strained because one side of your body is being overworked. This will frequently lead to back and neck pains.

• About food: In general, be very light on sugar products and eat plenty of fruits and vegetables. Cut down on your fat and salt intake. Eat more chicken and fish than red meat. Choose wholegrain breads rather than white breads.

• Exercising daily improves your metabolism. In fact, hours after exercising your body continues to burn more calories per minute than it did before that period of exercise. And it's true: on a fit body, the occasional splurge doesn't have nearly the impact that it has on an inactive, out-of-shape body. But if you're serious about losing weight, don't overeat or eat back the calories you burned off while exercising. (Depending on your size, weight, age, and how vigorously you do the exercises of the wind-up, the day's or days' sessions and the wind-down, you can burn up to 150 calories every fifteen minutes. But no matter how active you are, if you eat more than your energy expenditure, you will gain weight.

• To avoid straining your back, bend your knees and pull in your abdominal muscles toward your spine as you bend over to pick something up.

• Eat calmly whether you're by yourself or with others.

• Take your time. Rest your mind from problems; mental exhaustion, like physical exhaustion, leads to lower productivity and a shorter life span.

• Know what you're eating. Is it good for you or is it making you fat and slow?

• Enjoy the people you're around. Be active rather than passive; get involved.

• Be on time for meetings, appointments, and dates. Nervousness and anxiety can come from being late.

• When you're at work, if it's at all possible, call a friend, your husband, wife. Keep in touch with someone you love.

• If you don't like your job, find another one. If that's either too difficult or impossible to accomplish for one reason or another, make the rest of your day and life better. Follow the French Riviera Body Program, of course, and other activities, too, so you can better tolerate the part of your life that you don't fully enjoy.

• Make your life more creative. Write, draw, sing, read, go to the theater; channel your energy into whatever can make you the happiest, healthiest, and most attractive person. You will then reflect your contentment and energy, and inspire others to respond more positively toward you, and toward themselves, too.

• Make new friends, especially with those who share your exercising interests and enthusiasm. It makes it so much easier to stay on any fitness program, including this one, if you do.

• Show off your French Riviera Body. Apply your make-up properly. Attend to your hair, skin, and nails. Wear flattering colors and cuts of shoes and clothes. Choose clothes that fit well. Now that you're on the French Riviera Body Program you'll always be in shape, so you don't have to be concerned about whether or not your clothes will fit the next time you put them on.

Chapter 5

ANSWERS TO QUESTIONS

Here are answers to questions you may have about yourself and the French Riviera Body Program.

"I've never exercised before and I'm sixty years old. Is it too late for me to undertake the French Riviera Body Program?" "But I'm lazy. How do I make myself do it? I've never been able to stay on any self-improvement program. Help!" "I don't need to lose weight. I just want to firm up. Can I do this on the French Riviera Body Program?" "I belong to a health club. Why do I need the French Riviera Body Program?" "I'd like to exercise in the morning—that's when it's most convenient for me—but I wake up so stiff and tired. What should I do?" These questions and many more are answered here.

This chapter will also answer some age-old exercise questions like, "Will exercise make me tired?" "Will I get hungry from exercising?" "Should I expect to lose pounds or just inches?" "How much should I exercise?" "If I exercise a lot can I eat whatever I want? Can I eat extra desserts since I'm burning more calories?" and "Will exercise improve my sex life?"

Don't skip this chapter. Read it before you start this program.

Q. *What's the best sport or exercise to do for fitness?*
A. The one you enjoy is the best because that's the one you will continue to do. But the one you can do at least once a day is the most practical because it's essential to have a regular regimen to increase and preserve your strength, agility, and endurance.

Q. *Is the French Riviera Body Program just for young people?*
A. No. This program was created for all people regardless of age, strength, or flexibility. But I do insist that everyone check with a personal physician before starting this program or any other exercise program. Your doctor can advise you as to how long you should exercise each day and which exercises, if any, to omit because of a special limitation or handicap you may have.

Q. *I've never exercised before and I'm sixty years old. Is it too late for me to undertake the French Riviera Body Program?*
A. It's never too late to start taking better care of yourself. (Of course, like anybody else, you should check with your doctor and discuss this program with him or her before you start it.) People of any age can help themselves feel and look better by exercising and eating properly.

Always remember, your age is just a number. Old age or youthfulness can prevail at age eighteen or eighty-five. When the body is stiff and flabby, it feels and looks old; when it's exercised daily it can look and feel rejuvenated.

Sixty years old is as young or old as you want it to be.

Q. *I have arthritis. Can I exercise?*
A. Your doctor knows you better than I do, so he or she could answer you best. I can tell you about people with arthritis whom I have taught or interviewed: they all feel and look better when they exercise. By exercising they enjoy greater mobility in their joints, more resilience in their muscles,

and the strength and energy needed to carry out their daily activities. And they know that, by continuing a regular regimen of exercising, they can reduce and even prevent much of the disability that normally results from arthritis. Exercising makes living worthwhile.

Q. *Will I get hungry from exercising?*
A. Exercising will not make you hungrier than you usually are; in fact, it has been medically proven that exercise can help you develop your will power and can be an aid in the suppression of appetite.

Many people say that they have more control over how much they eat because exercising releases tension and stress; they don't react as impulsively or compulsively toward food. And because they're more conscious about their bodies, they are more determined and motivated to treat themselves right, by eating the kinds of food that support their exercise goals and achievements.

Q. *Will exercise make me tired?*
A. First of all, I am not suggesting that you exercise to the point of exhaustion. This program wasn't designed to tire you. *Au contraire*, I designed it to increase your level of energy on a daily basis for a lifetime.

Exercising to the point of mild fatigue is fine, even healthy. As you get stronger, more flexible and well-toned, you'll notice how your ability to exercise for longer periods of time without feeling even mildly fatigued increases. But, as you begin any exercise program, take it easy; don't overdo it.

The French Riviera Body Program is a beginning, not an end. It originated in a land where the sun's rays are direct, its effect enervating, and the importance of conserving one's energy consequently paramount. So follow this program as it is. Work hard, but don't knock yourself out. Let my exercises improve your life as they mold your body into the French Riviera Body.

Q. *Is this program safe for everyone?*
A. This program was designed for men and women in normal health and at any level of fitness. However, I recommend that everyone, especially those individuals with health problems and pregnant women, get the approval of their personal physician before they start.

Q. *Should I wear a bra to exercise?*
A. If you are more than a size B, I suggest you wear a bra to avoid straining the breast tissues.

Q. *When is the best time to exercise?*
A. The best time is whenever you make the time: morning, evening, or afternoon. The French Riviera Body 5-Minute, 7-Day Exercise Sessions in the morning can wake up your body; in the afternoon, they can refresh and revitalize you; and in the evening, they can release tension and stress while restoring your energy.

Q. *Can my children join me while I exercise?*
A. Of course! It's never too soon to develop a strong and flexible body and the habit of exercising.

Q. *I work in an office and I'm sitting all day, yet I'm ready to collapse when I get home from work. How can I start exercising when I can barely get myself together to prepare dinner?*
A. Oh boy! Do you need to exercise on the French Riviera Body Program! Sitting all day constricts your circulation which, in turn, reduces your energy level. It is natural that you feel that exercising is just about the last thing you can handle at the end of the day. Much of what you are experiencing as exhaustion also stems from inactivity, stress, and, possibly, lack of creative stimulation.

Let's change that. Now, you can create the French Riviera Body and exercise lifestyle for yourself, easily and conveniently, and maintain it for a lifetime.

Stimulate and challenge your body and mind with the French Riviera Body Program several times a day, once you're used to this program. For example, exercise before you go to work, during your lunch break, and as soon as you come home from work—before you take out the pots and pans, before you read your mail, before you answer the phone, put your bag down, take your coat off, and follow this program. It will revitalize your senses and refresh your body so you can do what you want to or have to do for the rest of the evening.

Invest five, ten, fifteen minutes or more each exercise period and you'll be rewarded with much more than energy and a shapely body. You'll find yourself feeling and looking happier, more productive, healthier, attractive, and optimistic.

Q. *Will exercise make me musclebound?*
A. Not the French Riviera Body Program's exercises. Having been a dancer, I have always been especially concerned with building strength, flexibility, and endurance into shapely, graceful muscles. My fitness-packed exercises concentrate on lengthening and elongating the line of your body for a beautiful, sleek look. As you follow this program you won't just look as if you're "in shape" with firm muscles and agile joints, you'll be working toward your best proportions and figure. Best of all, you'll soon be there.

Q. *But I'm lazy. How do I make myself do it? I've never been able to stay on any self-improvement program. Help!*
A. Take it easy. I know about being lazy and the trouble with staying on a program. That's why you're going to be able to follow the French Riviera Body Program and not allow laziness to get in the way of achieving the French Riviera Body.

Take my advice in "Special Tips": make several copies of the lead-off page to the French Riviera Body 5-Minute, 7-Day Exercise Sessions and the chart. Place them at various locations to remind yourself to follow this program. Fill in the chart with your schedule. Determine when, where, and with whom you will do the sessions. Try to pick the most practical times and places to do your exercises, otherwise, following this program will become an inconvenience, and ultimately, a goal you can't achieve. Keep this book with you at all times. And when the time and the place coincide, you'll be ready to follow the appropriate day's or days' sessions.

Think of exercising as a healthy habit, like brushing your teeth. You brush your teeth whether you like to or not because you know your teeth will decay if you don't and you know your teeth will look and feel better if you do. You also look and feel better when you exercise; and if you don't, your body looks and feels "horrible."

Be lazy about something you don't need, like preparing those late-night, calorie-packed snacks!

Never give yourself a choice. Don't make exercising an issue to consider; just do it and soon exercising will become a daily habit, a part of your life.

Q. *I have varicose veins. Is it safe to exercise?*
A. As a rule, check with your personal physician about any medical problems. I can only generalize.

In my experience, I have found that exercising can minimize and help prevent varicose veins. Active muscles will contribute to the easy flow of blood back to the heart. Restricted blood flow can cause the veins to bulge and ache.

Q. *I don't need to lose weight. I just want to firm up. Can I do this on the French Riviera Body Program?*
A. You can definitely firm up on the French Riviera Body Program. If you don't want to lose weight, adjust your calorie intake accordingly; eat a little more to replace the calories you expend as you exercise.

Q. *Can I exercise when it's very hot?*
A. Generally speaking, yes, especially if you have an air conditioner or fan. But on very hot days let your common sense—the way you feel and how you've reacted in the past to being physically active in hot weather—help you decide. Check with your doctor, too. If you have any medical problems that could be aggravated by exercising in hot weather, your doctor should be able to tell you.

Q. *Will exercise make my breasts bigger?*
A. For obvious reasons, I'm not asked this question too often. Exercise will not actually increase the size of your breasts, but your chest muscles will become much stronger and firmer, giving your breasts a higher, firmer, and shapelier appearance.

Q. *I really think I already get all the physical activity I need: I go bowling; I play golf; I have a job which requires me to stand most of the day; and I do my own housework. Do I need to follow the French Riviera Body Program?*
A. There are many benefits besides the physical ones that you can experience, enjoy, and put to good use by simply following this program. Exercising on this program isn't just a matter of doing exercises to look terrific, it's the creation of a new image—the new you—a feeling of vitality and an exercise lifestyle conducive to good health, productivity, and happiness.

Q. *I'm pregnant. Can I follow the French Riviera Body Program?*
A. *Please* ask your doctor! Every body is different and each pregnancy is unique. Pregnant women can follow this program but *doucement*

(gently, slowly)! Baby yourself a little. When you don't feel up to exercising, don't exercise. When you find an exercise is too difficult or uncomfortable to do, skip it.

Enjoy your pregnancy by following this program as best as you can. Being pregnant is a very special time of your life and exercising can help make your pregnancy even better. It can help you keep your energy level up and your strength, stamina, flexibility, and muscle tone "in shape." After you have your baby, you won't have such a big job ahead of you to get back in shape. You can concentrate more on your baby and less on those inches you must lose.

Q. *I'm on medication that makes me drowsy. Can I follow this program?*
A. Consult your prescribing physician. He or she knows you best, what you're taking, and how you should proceed with your activities, including the French Riviera Body Program.

Q. *Guess what? I'm too skinny; in fact, I have trouble putting on weight. Will exercising make me skinnier?*
A. Exercising has a moderating effect. It makes you feel and look stronger and more shapely as you improve your figure, muscle tone, flexibility, and endurance.

Like anyone else starting this program, first have a medical check-up. Make sure your "skinniness" isn't due to any unusual physical or emotional problem.

Q. *Why do I need to be in such good shape all year? The only time anyone really sees my body is during summer at the beach.*
A. If you don't care about your appearance during the winter, spring, or fall, then exercise for your health, enjoyment, relaxation, and youthfulness. Exercising is a wonderful anti-aging medicine, but only if you do it on a regular basis, all year round.

Getting in shape for the summer does not assure you of good physical fitness or a youthful life. You may look all right in your swimsuit but we both know it's only temporary. You need to exercise all year long; you need your body every day for work and play. And your body needs you—your attention and care—to be able to respond to your demands and requests, to withstand life's sudden crises, to preserve its shape and ability to function.

Good health and attractiveness are the results of eating and exercising consistently and correctly. Feeling great and looking terrific—having the French Riviera Body—shouldn't be a once-a-year phenomenon. It is *not* like a swimsuit; it's not something to slip on and off with the weather. Your body ought to be in good shape all year long!

Be ready for all life has in store, any time. You never know—you may win a trip, or want to treat yourself to a beach resort even during the winter. You can feel and look fabulous all year just by following this program. You'll look and feel at least twice as good as you would doing a crash course exercise program.

Q. *A lot of people talk about feeling exhilarated and euphoric from exercising. How soon will I feel that after I start this program?*
A. Moving the body in so many ways and getting the blood circulating briskly feels wonderful right from the start.

Q. *Should I expect to lose pounds or just inches?*
A. You will lose unwanted inches whether or not you lose weight. If you eat as you usually do or less, you will lose pounds, too.

Q. *How much should I exercise?*
A. Your present level of fitness, your age, occupation, lifestyle, health, the climate and altitude at which you live, and the goals you have are some determining factors. As a rule, you need enough exercise to keep your body and mind healthy, active, and happy and to accomplish your own personal fitness objectives. That means you may need and want to exercise for fifteen minutes once or twice a day—once you become accustomed to this program—whereas another person may want and need to exercise for forty minutes a day. Because it's such an individual matter and because each person responds to exercise at a different rate, it's best to see what exercising for X amount of time does for you. The right amount should make you feel energetic. (Of course, you may feel slightly tired immediately after exercising, but you should recover quickly.)

Remember! The French Riviera Body Program is not a contest. No one is judging you or competing with you. Be sensible: don't overexercise. Suffering isn't necessary; pain and exhaustion are not elements of this program. But don't be timid: if you underexercise (exercise less than the required five minutes without mitigating circumstances, like a recent illness), you'll only delay achievement of your goal, the French Riviera Body.

Q. *Can I exercise when I have my period?*
A. Generally speaking, yes. Most people find that exercising often relieves the cramps, tension, irritability, headaches, backaches, and bloatedness associated with menstruating.

Q. *Can I exercise before I go to bed or will exercising keep me awake?*
A. For some people, exercising just before bed-time is too invigorating; for others, it releases so much of their tension, stress, and imprisoned energy that sleeping is easy subsequently. You'll have to try it for yourself.

Q. *If I exercise a lot, can I eat whatever I want? Can I eat extra desserts since I'm burning more calories?*
A. It's true that by following this program of daily exercise you will increase the amount of muscle tissue in your body, making you more efficient at burning calories. Unlike fat, muscle tissue utilizes more calories to sustain itself even at rest so your metabolic rate goes up and stays up even after you exercise. So, if you exercise and diet, you'll have an easier time maintaining your ideal weight or losing weight.

But if you don't want to gain weight and you want to stay well, have lots of energy, and live a long time, it's wise not to overeat, especially those sugar snacks and desserts.

Q. *I have a cold. Should I exercise?*
A. With a simple cold—runny nose, stuffy head—it's okay to exercise. Many people do. However, if you have a fever, I recommend that you do not exercise, since exercising increases your internal body temperature. Instead, get some rest and when you feel better, return to this program gradually.

Q. *Will exercise improve my sex life?*
A. It most positively can! Exercise improves the body physically and mentally. You will become more secure about your own body, more comfortable with yourself. As a whole, you will be much more attractive to others than you ever thought possible.

Q. *I belong to a health club. Why do I need the French Riviera Body Program?*
A. Belonging to a health club and exercising there regularly are two different stories. I know, and I'll bet you do, too, many people who belong to health clubs, go there a few times and never again. But regardless of whether or not you fall into that group or the group who actually makes use of a health club, this program can do you so much good that I have to answer your question by saying, Yes! You need to follow the French Riviera Body Program.

Q. *I've just spent six weeks convalescing from an illness. How should I begin this program?*
A. First ask your doctor when you can start. Then start as I instruct those who have never exercised before or are extremely out of shape to begin.

The key to recovering successfully from an illness is to realize that you have been ill, that you are probably weaker now than you were, and that returning to your usual activities and new ones requires patience and understanding toward your body. So don't panic and don't rush! Be nice to yourself: work into this program gradually and you will not only regain but will surpass your former strength, flexibility, and stamina.

Q. *How fast or slowly should I do the exercises?*
A. There isn't any fixed rule as to the pace at which the exercises should be done. Vary the speed and let the way you breathe—how fast or slow—guide you. In addition, of course, you should always take your present condition and age into account.

Q. *I'd like to exercise in the morning—that's when it's most convenient for me—but I wake up so stiff and tired. What should I do?*
A. Wake up slowly by doing some of the preliminary wind-ups in bed. (Those that are adaptable have been designated by a ✓.) Get out of bed at a leisurely pace and continue with the additional wind-ups. Turn to the day's session and do each exercise without pushing, straining, or rushing. (If you are following the St. Tropez Body Plan, follow each of the two consecutive days' sessions from wind-up to wind-down.) Breathe deeply. Go slowly. Take a bath or shower to loosen up your muscles and joints. Then, once you're used to the program and it's convenient, do another period of exercise at a brisker pace.

Q. *I have cellulite. Should I have special treatments to get rid of it?*
A. The American Medical Association has determined that those so-called miracle devices and treatments to eliminate cellulite are nothing more than a hoax.

Cellulite is simply fat. By following this program exactly as described you will reduce or eliminate your cellulite. You—and not some device—will be burning your fat away.

Q. *I've never exercised before. Will I be sore the next day? And if I am, should I do that day's session?*
A. Since you've never exercised before, start this program very slowly. Follow my instructions in the "Basic Rules." Should you become sore, continue to follow this program anyway. Take warm baths, too. As your body gets used to exercising, the soreness will disappear.

THE BENEFITS OF THE FRENCH RIVIERA BODY PROGRAM
5-MINUTE • 7-DAY EXERCISE SESSIONS

Develops a feeling of pride in yourself

Improves your posture

Helps you think clearer and faster

Corrects your body alignment

Boosts your morale and confidence

Makes you sexier, stronger, more coordinated, flexible, graceful, and energetic

Trims and shapes your waist, hips, thighs, buttocks, calves, ankles, upper arms, and abdomen

Enhances your ability and performance in other activities

Improves the capacity of your heart, lungs, and circulatory system

Eliminates and prevents back and neck pains

Increases your stamina

Contributes to healthier looking and feeling hair and skin

Reduces the need to diet

Burns fat and calories

Releases physical and emotional stress, anxiety, and tension

Gives you a look of authority and power

Helps you lose weight and inches; helps you stay at your ideal weight

Reduces and eliminates headaches

Contributes to better relationships and more productivity at home and at work

Improves your digestion

Helps you look and feel years younger

Firms and tones sagging and flabby muscles

Promotes discipline so you set goals and reach them

Helps you look and feel glamorous, chic, calm, dynamic, radiant, sleek, elegant, and healthy

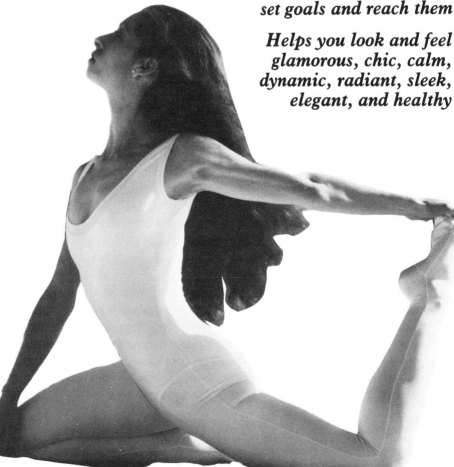

27

Chapter 6

THE WIND-UP
• AND •
THE WIND-DOWN

These wind-up exercises will prepare you for your day's session by speeding up your heart rate, releasing tension and stress, loosening sluggish and stiff joints, increasing blood circulation, raising your body temperature, and stretching and toning your ligaments, muscles, and connective tissues so you will get the most out of your time and energy—and this program. You will do the exercises with greater ease and better results.

Do these exercises before you begin each day's session!

Here are some quick preliminary wind-up exercises that you can do either sitting or standing. Those marked with a ✓ can also be done while you're still in bed.

Pull your abdominal muscles in toward your back and up toward your ribs. Tighten your buttocks. Let's go. . . .

1. Move your head in a circle: Tilt your head over your right shoulder. Roll your head back lifting your chin toward the ceiling. When your head is over your left shoulder, roll your head forward, lowering your chin to your chest. When your head reaches your right shoulder again, reverse the circle.

✓2. Move your shoulders in a circle: Pull your shoulders forward. Lift them up toward your ears. Bring them back. Then pull them down. Reverse the circle: Pull your shoulders back. Lift them up toward your ears. Bring them forward. Then pull them down.

✓3. Spread your fingers apart, then close your hands into tight fists.

✓4. With your hands in tight fists, move your wrists in circles to the right, then to the left.

✓5. Move your arms in a circle: Bring your arms forward, perpendicular to your body. Raise them over your head. Pull them back as far as you can. Then bring them to your sides. Reverse the circle: Pull your arms back. Raise them over your head. Then bring them back to the forward position, and finally to your sides again.

✓6. Curl your toes, then stretch and flex them.

✓7. Move your feet and ankles in circles to the right and to the left.

✓8. Hold your right knee with both hands. Then press your knee toward your chest and touch it with your forehead. Do the same with your left knee.

Exercises 9-14: Great for releasing tension from your face and jaw and for toning up your chin and facial muscles.

✓9. Open your mouth wide and then close it.

✓10. Roll your eyes to the right, then to the left.

✓11. Lift your eyebrows toward your hairline, then pull them down toward your nose.

✓12. Open your eyes wide, then close them tight.

✓13. Puff up your cheeks, then let the air out.

✓14. Pucker your mouth, then smile.

Now stand up (if you're not already up) to do the following wind-ups.

WIND-UP

Preparatory Position: *Get Ready!*

Stand erect with your feet placed a bit wider than shoulder-distance apart. Turn your legs slightly to the outside: Turn your right foot toward the right side and your left foot toward the left side. Then extend your arms forward at shoulder level. Turn the palms of your hands down. Flex your hands back at the wrists, then, rotating your wrists, point your fingers toward each other. Pull in your abdominal muscles toward your back and up toward your ribs. Tighten your buttocks. Pull your shoulders back and down. Hold your chin and chest high. Let's go!

1a. Breathe in as you rise up onto the balls of your feet. Stretch your arms directly overhead, flexing your hands back at the wrists and pointing your fingers in toward each other. Don't bend your knees or elbows or separate your arms. Pull in your abdominal muscles and tighten your buttocks. Don't hunch your shoulders, pull them back and down. Hold your chin and chest high. Stretch your whole body upward. Then . . .

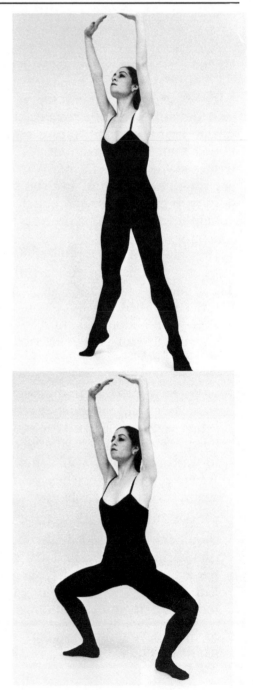

1b. Breathe out as you lower your heels to the floor. Bend your knees. Don't move your arms. Tighten your abdominal muscles and buttocks. Keep your shoulders back and down, your chin and chest high and your back straight. Now . . .

30

1c. Breathe in as you bend forward from your hips. Don't move your arms. Keep your back straight. Reach your upper back and buttocks toward the ceiling and your waist toward the floor. Hold your chin and chest high. Straighten your knees. Don't move your feet. Pull in your abdominal muscles. Tighten your buttocks. Then . . .

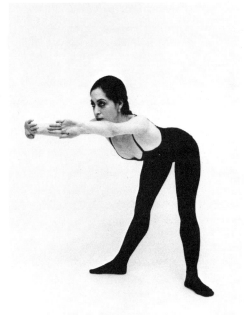

1d. Breathe out as you again bend your knees. Don't lift your heels off the floor. Lower your head, aiming your chin toward your chest. Reach your buttocks and chest toward the floor and your waist toward the ceiling. Don't move your arms. Now roll slowly through each vertebra to stand upright. Keep your knees bent, your head down, your abdominal muscles pulled in and your buttocks tight.

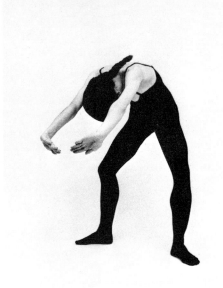

Don't repeat. Remain standing for the next exercise.

Preparatory Position: *Get Ready!*

Standing, with your legs placed wider than shoulder-distance apart and turned slightly to the outside, extend your arms forward with the palms of your hands facing down. Pull your abdominal muscles in toward your back and up toward your ribs. Tighten your buttocks. Pull your shoulders back and down. Hold your chin and chest high. Stretch up each vertebra, increasing the space between your hips and ribs. Let's go!

2a. Breathe in as you raise your arms overhead. Spread your fingers apart. Rise up on the balls of your feet. Keep your knees and elbows straight. Lift your chin and chest upward. Pull in your abdominal muscles and tighten your buttocks. Pull your weight up out of your torso. Then . . .

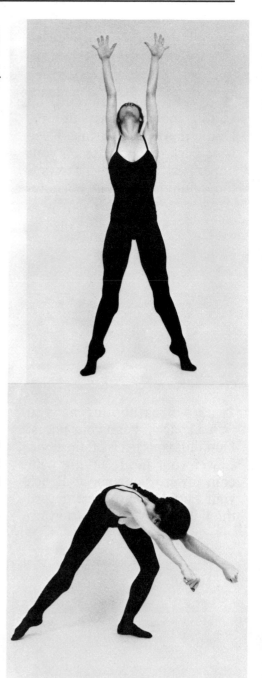

2b. Breathe out as you close your fingers into tight fists. Shift your weight onto your left foot and press your left heel to the floor. Bend your left knee. Straighten your right knee and point your right foot. Bend forward toward the left side. Now . . .

2c. Shift your weight onto your right foot and press your right heel to the floor. Bend your right knee. Swing your torso and arms to the right side. Keep your elbows straight and your fingers closed into tight fists. Straighten your left knee and point your left foot. Pull in your abdominal muscles and tighten your buttocks. Then straighten up your back. Stand erect with both feet flat on the floor.

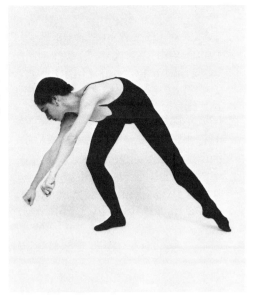

Repeat once, circling the other way. Then start today's session. If you're on the St. Tropez Body plan and you've already done today's session, do tomorrow's.

WIND-DOWN

After the wind-ups and the day's session, it's essential to cool down since your blood is pumping rapidly throughout your body. An important component of the French Riviera Body Program, the wind-down helps circulate blood back to your heart. This exercise gives you a chance to relax and recharge. It makes you feel great, in control, and ready to go.

Preparatory Position: *Get Ready!*

Stand erect with your feet placed a little wider than shoulder-distance apart and pointing forward. Pull in your abdominal muscles toward your back and up toward your ribs. Tighten your buttocks. Pull your shoulders back and down. Hold your chin and chest high. Pull your weight up off your hips, increasing the space between your hips and ribs. Relax your arms at your sides. Let's go!

3a. Breathe in as you raise your arms over your head. Turn the palms of your hands forward. Rise up onto the balls of your feet. Stretch your whole body upward. Pull in your abdominal muscles. Tighten your buttocks. Hold your chin and chest high. Pull your shoulders back and down. Stretch your fingers, knees, and elbows. (Incline your weight slightly forward over your toes to help you balance.) Then . . .

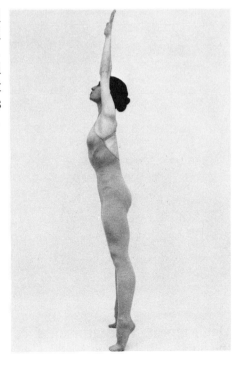

3b. Breathe out as you put your heels on the floor. Bend your knees. Lower your head, aiming your chin toward your chest. Count to 16 as you roll through each vertebra bending forward. (Close your eyes: Think of peaceful and beautiful things. Fantasize and daydream if you wish. Let go of your tension, stress, and nervousness. Bring in new energy.) Pull your abdominal muscles in and tighten your buttocks. Relax your toes, ankles, neck, shoulders, face, arms, hands, fingers, and back. Don't come up yet! Stay down and breathe normally. Turn your head from side to side. Lift and lower your shoulders, then move them around in a circle. Shake your hands and arms. Now take in a deep breath.

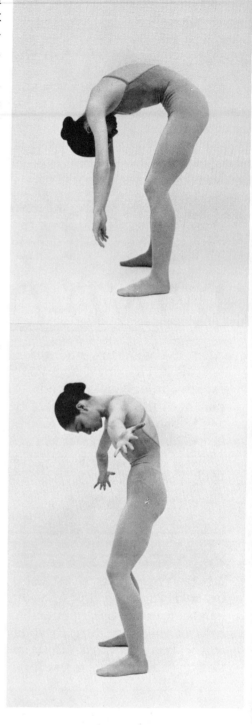

3c. Breathe out as—counting to 16—you roll up through each vertebra into position #3a: Keep your knees bent. Incline your chin toward your chest. Pull your abdominal muscles in. Tighten your buttocks. Relax your neck, shoulders, back, face, feet, ankles, and toes. Stretch your arms out to the sides, then lift them over your head. Spread your fingers apart. Lift your chin and chest. Straighten your knees and rise onto the balls of your feet.

Don't repeat. To continue exercising, begin with the wind-ups on page 30.

Chapter 7

THE 5 • MINUTE, 7 • DAY
EXERCISE SESSIONS

Before we do Monday's session let's warm up with the exercises in the wind-up section on pages 29–33.

Preparatory Position: *Get Ready!*

Stand erect with your feet positioned a little wider than hip-distance apart and pointing straight forward. Distribute your weight equally on both legs and lean slightly forward over your toes; be light on your heels. Pull your abdominal muscles in toward your back and up toward your ribs. Stretch your body upward from your hips through your ribs to your collarbone and the middle of your head. Tighten your buttock muscles. Pull your shoulders back and down. Hold your chin and chest high. Now place your fingertips on top of your shoulders. Lift your elbows above shoulder level and aim them sideways. Bend your knees. Don't lift your heels off the floor. Let's go!

1a. Breathe in as you straighten your knees. Pull your elbows and shoulders back. Lift your chin and chest upward. Don't drop your elbows lower than shoulder height. Pull in your abdominal muscles and tighten your buttocks. Then . . .

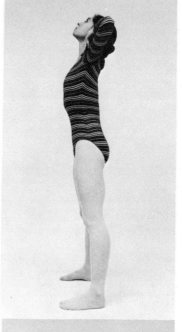

1b. Breathe out as you bend your knees. Keep your heels on the floor. Bring your elbows together in front of your face. Lower your head, aiming your chin toward your chest and bend forward at the waist, curving your upper back. Pull your abdominal muscles in and tighten your buttocks. Relax your face, neck, and shoulders.

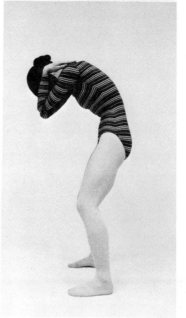

Repeat twice. Remain standing to do the next exercise.

MONDAY

Preparatory Position: *Get Ready!*

Bend your knees and keep your back straight. Don't tilt your pelvis forward or backward. (Your hips should be in line with your shoulders). Remember your abdominal and buttocks muscles! Stretch your spine by pulling your weight up out of your torso; feel the distance between your hips and ribs increase. Hold your chin and chest high. Now place the fingertips of your left hand on top of your left shoulder and lift your left elbow to shoulder level. Raise your right arm over your head, bringing it close to your right ear. Turn the palm of your right hand to the left side. Let's go!

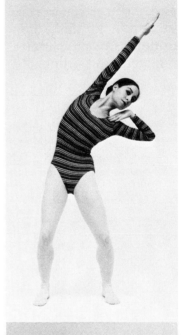

2a. Breathe in as you stretch your body upward, then bend at the waist toward your left side, tilting your head over your left shoulder. Don't straighten your knees. Keep your left elbow raised. Pull your shoulders down and back. (Give special attention to keeping your right shoulder back and your right arm close to your right ear.) Pull in your abdominal muscles and tighten your buttocks. Keep your heels on the floor. Hold your chin and chest high. Then . . .

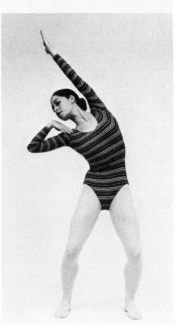

2b. Breathe out as you place the fingertips of your right hand on top of your right shoulder. Lift your right elbow to shoulder level and extend your left arm over your head, bringing it close to your left ear. Turn the palm of your left hand to the right side. Then stretch your body upward and bend at the waist to the right side, tilting your head over your right shoulder. Keep your knees bent, your heels on the floor, and your shoulders down and back. (Give special attention to keeping your left shoulder back and your left arm close to your left ear.) Remember your abdominal muscles and buttocks! Hold your chin and chest high.

Repeat twice vigorously. Remain standing to do the next exercise.

Preparatory Position: *Get Ready!*

As you stand with your feet facing forward, positioned a little wider than hip-distance apart, stretch your knees. Raise your arms over your head with the palms of your hands facing forward. Now bend forward from your hips without bending your back or your knees. (But if the backs of your legs are too stiff or out of shape, modify this position; bend your knees.) Stretch your back from the base of your spine through the tips of your fingers. Pull your abdominal muscles in toward your back and up toward your ribs. Tighten your buttocks. Let's go!

3a. Breathe in as you arrive at and hold this "flat back" position. Stretch your elbows and fingers. Lift your chin and look past your hands. Tighten your abdominals and buttocks and then . . .

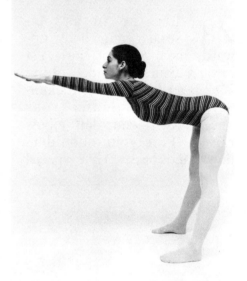

3b. Breathe out as you bend your knees. Lower your head, aiming your chin toward your chest. Then curve your spine by pulling in your abdominal muscles extra tightly and pushing the middle of your back toward the ceiling and your buttocks and head down toward the floor. Point your hands downward at an angle to maintain the curve of your torso. Don't drop your arms; position them by your ears. Relax your face and neck. Keep your buttocks tight and your heels on the floor.

Don't stand up yet!

To return to 3a, stretch the middle of your back down toward the floor and your buttocks and head up toward the ceiling. Straighten your knees.

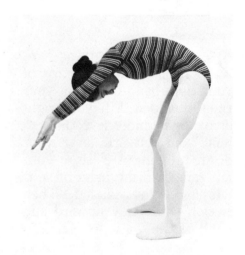

Repeat twice fluidly. Stand up slowly. Now turn to exercise #4.

MONDAY

Preparatory Position: *Get Ready!*

Stand with your legs together, distributing your weight equally on both feet. Stretch your arms down by your sides with the palms of your hands facing back. Stretch your fingers and keep them together. Then flex your hands back at the wrists.

Pull your shoulders back and down. Now bend your knees. Pull in your abdominal muscles toward your back and up toward your ribs. Tighten your buttocks, stretch your spine upward and hold your chin and chest high. Let's go!

4a. Breathe in as you lift your left foot, pointing it, next to your right knee, which should still be bent. Swing your arms straight forward to shoulder level with your hands still in a flexed position.

Don't separate your fingers or bend your elbows. Pull your weight up off your hips and tighten your abdominal and buttock muscles. Pull your shoulders back and down. Hold your chin and chest high. Then . . .

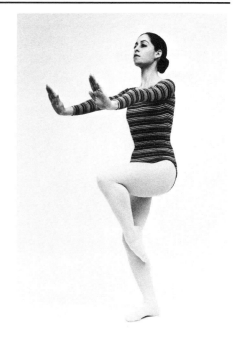

4b. Breathe out as you jump from your right foot to your left. Bend your left knee. Lift your right foot up, pointing it next to your left knee. Swing your arms straight back as far as possible. Keep your hands in a flexed position, your elbows and fingers straight, your abdominal and buttocks muscles tight, your chin and chest high and your shoulders back and down. Now return to 4a: Jump up from your left foot and land on your right foot. Bend your right knee.

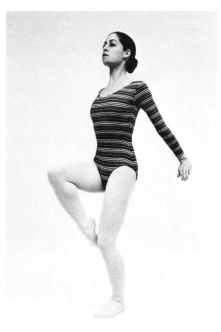

Repeat four times at a brisk and even pace. Then sit down for exercise #5.

Preparatory Position: *Get Ready!*

Sitting down, straighten your legs out in front of you. Point your feet. Interlace your fingers behind your back. (But if you have trouble with this arm position, modify it: place your hands on your hips and keep them there throughout this exercise.) Stretch through each vertebra from the base of your spine up to your neck; pull your weight up out of your buttocks and hips. Pull your abdominal muscles in and tighten your buttocks. Hold your chin and chest high. Pull your shoulders back and down. Let's go!

5a. Breathe in as you bend your elbows outward and touch your back with your hands. Pull your shoulders back and down. Lift your chin and chest. Flex your feet back at the ankles and straighten up your back. Don't bend your knees. Abdominal muscles in, buttocks tight. Stretch your torso upward. Then . . .

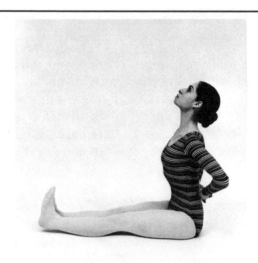

5b. Breathe out as you bend forward, aiming your forehead toward your legs. (But if at first it's too difficult to bend forward toward your legs with your knees straight, modify this position; bend forward with your knees bent.) Straighten your elbows, lifting your arms up behind your back. Don't separate your hands or bend your knees. Point your feet. Pull in your abdominal muscles! Relax your neck and face. Keep your shoulders back.

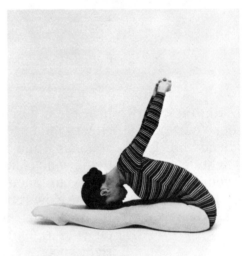

Repeat twice smoothly. Remain seated to do the next exercise.

Preparatory Position: *Get Ready!*

Sitting, spread your legs until you feel the pull along your inner thigh muscles. Keep your right leg straight out to the side and place the sole of your left foot next to the inside of your upper right thigh. Point your feet. Pull your abdominal muscles in toward your back and up toward your ribs. Stretch your spine upward. Let's go!

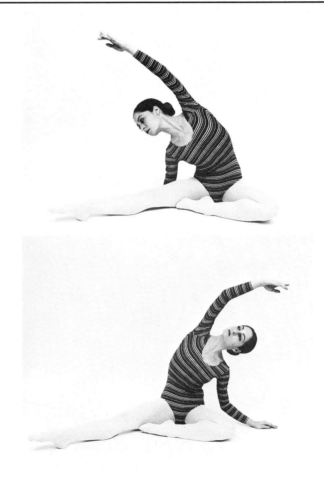

6a. Breathe in as you raise your left arm in a gentle curve over your head, with the palm of your hand facing right. Position your fingers gracefully. Place your right hand on the floor behind your right leg in alignment with your hips. Bend your right elbow toward your hips, then place it on the floor. Bend to the right side. Tilt your head over your right shoulder, stretching the left side of your neck. Don't move your legs. Pull your shoulders down and back, especially your left shoulder. Keep your left outer thigh aimed at the floor, your feet pointed, and your buttocks on the floor, especially the left side. Remember your abdominal and buttocks muscles! Hold your chin and chest high. Then . . .

6b. Breathe out as you push off your right hand and lift your right arm over your head. Again, your right arm should form a gentle curve with the palm of your hand facing left. Position your fingers gracefully. Pull your weight up and off your hips. Place your left hand on the floor out to the left side in alignment with your hips. Bend your left elbow toward your hips, then place it on the floor. Bend to the left side and tilt your head over your left shoulder, stretching the muscles in the right side of your neck. Don't twist your shoulders. Pull them down and back, especially your right shoulder. Don't move your legs, and keep your outer left thigh aimed at the floor, your feet pointed, and your buttocks on the floor, especially on the right side. Hold your chin and chest high. Tighten your buttocks and abdominal muscles.

Repeat twice at a quick pace. Then reverse to the opposite leg and arm positions and repeat the exercise. Remain seated to do exercise #7.

MONDAY

Preparatory Position: *Get Ready!*

Sit erect with your legs straight out in front of you. Bend your right knee, aiming your right outer thigh toward the floor, then place the heel of your right foot underneath the hamstring—the back of the thigh—of your left leg. At shoulder-distance apart with your fingers pointing forward, position your hands on the floor behind your torso. Remember your abdominal muscles and your buttocks. Straighten your back; feel the distance increase between your hips and ribs. Point your feet. (If at first this exercise is too difficult, modify it: do not lift your buttocks and outer thigh off the floor in part 7b. Just keep your leg lifted and bend and straighten your knee and elbows as directed.) Let's go!

7a. Breathe in as you bend your elbows, inclining your torso back. Bend your left knee to the outside, lifting it up toward your chest. Point your feet. Pull your shoulders back and down. Hold your chin and chest high. Tighten your abdominal and buttock muscles. Then . . .

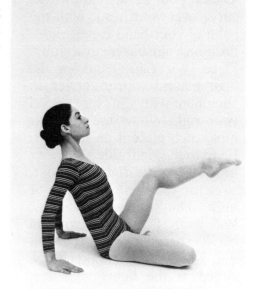

7b. Breathe out as you press down on the palms of your hands, stretching your elbows. Push forward and upward with your hips, raising your buttocks and outer right thigh off the floor. Straighten your left knee. Lift your left leg as high as you can, stretching your inner thigh and heel up. Tighten your buttocks. Pull your abdominal muscles in. Keep your back straight, your shoulders pulled back and down, your chin and chest high, and your feet pointed. Don't move your hands. Return to 7a: Bend your elbows. Lower your buttocks to the floor and bend your left knee.

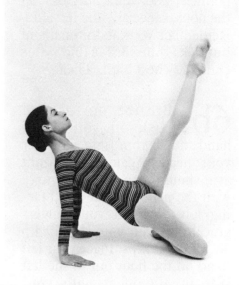

Repeat the exercise twice. Then reverse to do your other leg. Roll onto your left side for the next exercise.

*If you've never exercised before or are very much out of shape, omit this exercise the first week.

MONDAY

Preparatory Position: *Get Ready!*

Lying on your left side, support your torso by placing your left elbow to the side of your rib cage and your left hand in front of your left shoulder. Stretch your legs to the side in alignment with your shoulders, hips, and left elbow. Point your feet. Pull your shoulders back and down. Hold your chin and chest high. Keep the left side of your torso elevated by pushing down onto your left forearm and hand. Pull your abdominal muscles in toward your back. Tighten your buttock muscles. Slide your right knee along the floor and place it in front of your waist. Extend your right arm out to the side over your left leg. Turn the palm of your right hand down. Turn your head to the right. Keep your left leg straight. Let's go!

8a. Breathe in as you pull your right knee back, aiming your knee cap upward. Put your right hand flat on the floor in front of your waist. Place your right foot next to your left knee, pointing your toes toward the floor. Stretch your left leg out on the floor and point your left foot. Keep your abdominal muscles and buttocks tight, your shoulders back and down (especially your left one), and your head turned to the right. Push down onto your left forearm and hand to keep the upper left side of your body lifted off the floor. Hold your chin and chest high. Then . . .

8b. Breathe out as you push your right knee down toward the floor. Lift your left leg off the floor, keeping it in alignment with your hips, shoulders, and left elbow. Don't bend your left knee but remember to point your feet. With the palm of your right hand facing down, extend your right arm to the side over your raised leg. Position your fingers gracefully. Look past your right hand. Abdominal muscles in, buttocks tight. Pull your shoulders back and down, especially your left one.

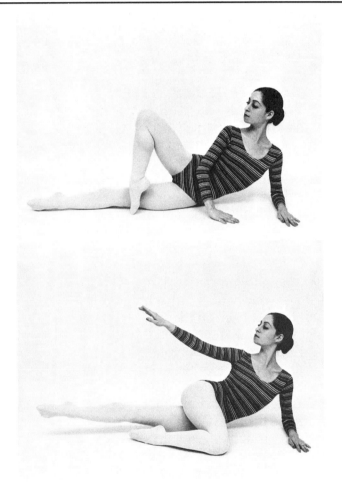

Hold your chin and chest high. Don't let your body sink to the floor. Push down onto your left forearm and hand to keep the left side of your body raised.

Repeat twice. Do the same exercises with your other leg. Then lie on your back to do exercise #9.

Preparatory Position: *Get Ready!*

Lying on your back, place your hands behind your head and interlace your fingers. Bend your knees. Slide your feet flat on the floor toward your buttocks, keeping your knees, ankles, and feet together. Press the small of your back to the floor. Pull your abdominal muscles down toward your back. Tighten your buttocks. Relax your neck, face, and shoulders. Let's go!

9a. Breathe in as you bring your knees toward your chest. Flex your feet back at the ankles. Position your feet lower than your knees. Rest your upper back, neck, elbows, and head on the floor. Incline your chin toward your chest. Pull your abdominal muscles down toward your back. Tighten your buttocks. Keep the small of your back on the floor and your knees, ankles, and feet together. Don't move your hands out of place. Then . . .

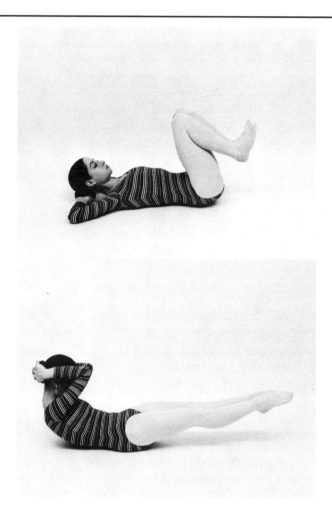

9b. Breathe out as you point your feet. With the help of your hands, lift your head and upper back off the floor aiming your chin toward your chest. Don't separate your fingers. Pull your elbows together in front of your forehead. Extend your legs forward to about 15″ from the floor. (But if it's too difficult to straighten your legs 15″ from the floor with the small of your back on the floor, modify this exercise: Straighten your legs at a higher level.) Buttocks and abdominal muscles! Press the small of your back to the floor. Then lower your upper back and head to the floor. Open your elbows and bend your knees toward your chest. Now you're ready to repeat 9a. (For a more intense abdominal workout, straighten your legs lower than 15″ above the floor. Be sure to keep the small of your back down on the floor at all times!)

Repeat twice, then roll onto your right side. Put both hands on the floor to help you sit up. Then go onto your hands and knees to do exercise #10.

Preparatory Position: *Get Ready!*

When you are on your hands and knees, put your knees together and place your hands directly underneath your shoulders, pointing your fingers forward. Distribute your weight equally between your hands and knees. Point your feet. Relax your neck and face. Pull your abdominal muscles up toward your spine. Tighten your buttocks. Slide your left foot back directly behind your left hip, then lift your left leg off the floor. Let's go!

10a. Breathe in as you bend your elbows with resistance. Lower your chest to the floor and aim your forehead in between your hands. Keep your back straight. Straighten your left knee and lower your left leg. Touch the floor with your left foot. Don't lean or tilt to either side. Pull your shoulders back and down. Keep your abdominal and buttocks muscles tight and your feet pointed. Then . . .

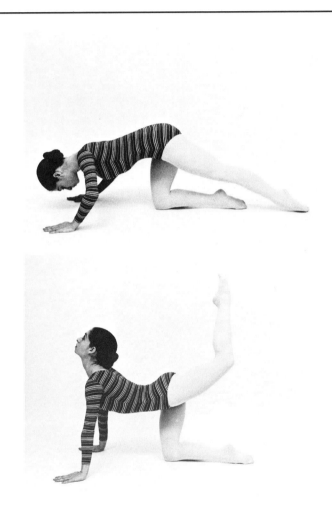

10b. Breathe out as you straighten your elbows with resistance by pushing down onto your hands. Raise your chest away from the floor. Lift your chin and left leg up smoothly. Bend your left knee, aiming your pointed foot to the ceiling. Don't let your left leg go out toward the side. Move it directly behind your left shoulder and hip. Don't change the position of your hands. Keep your feet pointed, your shoulders pulled down and back, your abdominals and buttocks tight, and your weight equally distributed between both hands. Look up at the ceiling.

Repeat twice. Do the same with your other leg. Then stand up slowly. Now turn to pages 33–34 for the wind-down.

TUESDAY

Let's warm-up a little. Turn to pages 29–33 for the wind-up exercises, then return to this page.

Preparatory Position: *Get Ready!*

Sit down and cross your legs Indian style. (But if you have enormous difficulty sitting Indian style, then sit with your legs straight out in front of you.) Pull your abdominal muscles in toward your back and up toward your ribs. Tighten your buttocks. Relax with your arms down at your sides. Stretch your spine straight and long; pull your weight up from your seat to the top of your head. Let's go!

1a. Breathe in as you raise your arms over your head with the palms of your hands facing each other. Stretch your fingers and keep them together. Reach up as high as you can, keeping your arms close to your head. Raise your chin and chest. Stretch each vertebra. Pull in and tighten . . . Then . . .

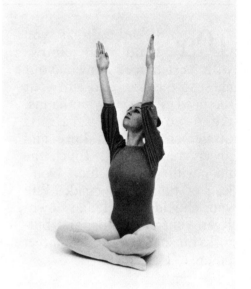

1b. Breathe out as you bend forward from your waist. Bring your arms down to the sides at shoulder level with your hands flexed back at the wrists. Keep your elbows straight and your fingers together. Lower your head, aiming your chin toward your chest. Tighten your buttocks but don't lift them off the floor. Pull your abdominal muscles in tight. Relax your neck and face.

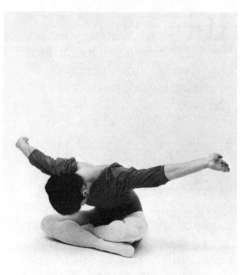

Repeat twice. Remain seated for exercise #2.

Preparatory Position: *Get Ready!*

Straighten your legs out in front of you and put your heels together. Rotate your legs to the outside. Tighten your abdominal and buttock muscles. Stretch each vertebra upward in a straight line. Interlace your fingers with the palms of your hands facing out. Now raise your arms above your head. Let's go!

2a. Breathe in as you lean back. Lower your arms to chest level. Keeping your elbows and knees straight and your fingers together, lower your chin toward your chest. Bring your shoulders forward, stretching your upper back. Then point your feet and bring them together, rotating your legs toward each other. Remember your buttock and abdominal muscles. But if it is too difficult for you to do this exercise as it is, modify it by bending your knees and/or your elbows. Then . . .

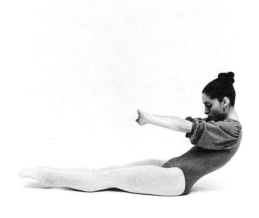

2b. Breathe out as you raise your arms over your head. Don't separate your hands or bend your elbows or knees. Incline your upper body forward over your legs with your back straight. Flex your feet back at the ankles. Rotate your legs slightly to the outside from your hips and aim your small toes at the floor. Pull your shoulders back and down. Lift your chin and chest. Tighten. . . .

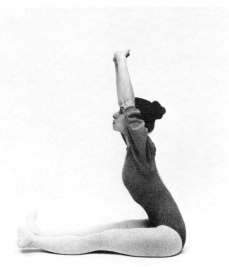

Repeat twice. Remain seated for the next exercise.

Preparatory Position: *Get Ready!*

As you sit, split your legs as far apart as you can without straining. Feel the pull along the insides of your legs—but if you're in pain bring your legs closer together. Pull in your abdominal muscles and tighten your buttocks. Lift your weight up from your seat, hips, and waist. Hold your chin and chest high. Now bring your arms up with the palms of your hands facing each other. Then point your fingers toward each other gracefully and form a circle around your head with your arms. Keep your shoulders down and back. Relax your neck. Let's go!

3a. Breathe in as you straighten your spine, pulling up off your hips and out of your torso. Tighten your buttocks and pull in your abdominal muscles. Straighten your knees. Stretch your legs along the floor. Point your feet. Turn your head to the right. Hold your chin and chest high. Keep your shoulders back and down, especially your left one. Then . . .

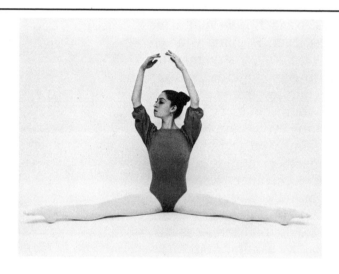

3b. Breathe out as you reach and bend to the right side. Don't lean forward or backward or twist to face your leg. Pull your shoulders back and down, especially your left one. Bend your knees up toward the ceiling. Flex your feet back at the ankles. Keep your buttocks on the floor (especially the left side.) Hold your chin and chest high. Don't change the position of your arms or hands. Continue the curve of your arms through your wrists and fingers. Look right toward your foot. Remember your abdominal and buttocks muscles.

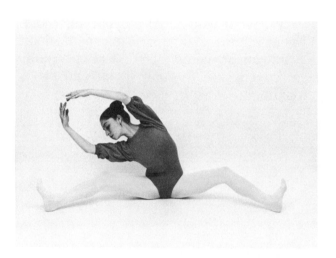

Repeat twice fluidly at a quick pace and follow the same routine for the other side. Then roll onto your right side for exercise #4.

TUESDAY

Preparatory Position: *Get Ready!*

Lying on your right side, position your right elbow out to the side of your rib cage and place your right hand flat on the floor facing forward. Pull in your abdominal muscles toward your back. Tighten your buttocks. Push down onto your right forearm and hand to keep the right side of your torso raised off the floor. Let's go!

4a. Breathe in as you stretch your legs together in alignment with your hips, shoulders, and right elbow. Keep your back straight and point your feet. Abdominal muscles in; tighten buttocks. Stretch your left arm forward in front of your left shoulder. Turn the palm of your left hand down. Position your fingers gracefully and look past them. Keep both shoulders back and down, particularly your right one. Hold your chin and chest high. Don't sink down into your right side. Then . . .

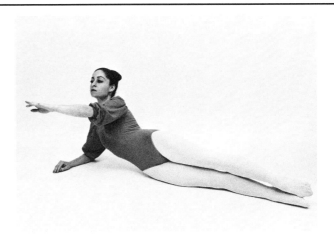

4b. Breathe out as you swing your left leg directly forward, your left foot flexed back at the ankle. Keep your right foot pointed. Swing your left arm to the left side at shoulder level. Flex your left hand back at the wrist. Stretch your left elbow. Keep your knees straight. Pull and tighten. . . . Don't rock your body, twist your shoulders, or move your right leg. Hold your chin and chest high. Be sure not to sink down to the floor on your right side or raise your right shoulder up toward your ear.

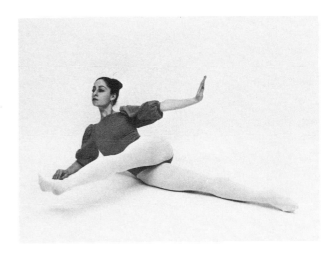

Repeat twice on each side. Then lie on your back for the next exercise.

Preparatory Position: *Get Ready!*

Lying on your back and keeping your tailbone on the floor, bring your knees up toward your chest. Pull your abdominal muscles down toward your back. Tighten your buttocks. Stretch your arms out to the sides at shoulder level with the palms of your hands facing down. Relax your neck, shoulders, fingers, face, and arms.

5a. Breathe in as you move your knees as close to your chest as possible with the small of your back still on the floor. Point your feet. Pull and tighten. . . . Incline your chin toward your chest. Look at your knees. Keep your neck, shoulders, fingers, face, and arms relaxed. Press your knees, ankles, and feet together. Then . . .

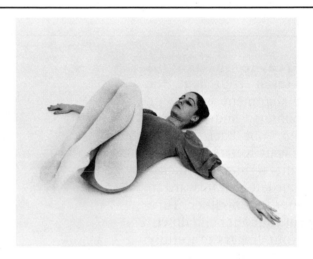

5b. Breathe out as you bring your knees directly over to the floor on the left side at waist level. Don't move your arms. Straighten your right knee only. Don't separate your legs; keep your inner thighs tight together. Touch the floor on the left side with your right foot. Turn your head to the right and look past your right hand. Pull and tighten. . . . And keep both shoulders on the floor, especially your right one. Point your feet. Then bend your right knee, bringing your ankles together. Move your knees toward your chest again and lie flat on your back.

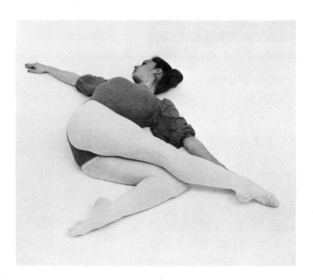

Repeat four times alternating sides. Stay on your back to do the next exercise.

TUESDAY

Preparatory Position: *Get Ready!*

Lying on your back, bend your knees and put your feet flat on the floor. (Bend your knees only slightly to facilitate this exercise. If you still have trouble sitting up all the way due to weak back and abdominal muscles, bring your hands together and lift only your head and upper back off the floor.) Let's go!

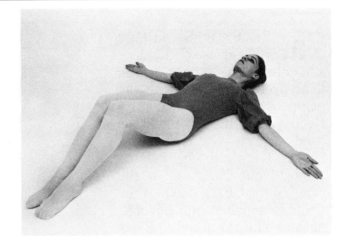

6a. Breathe in as you extend your arms out to the sides at shoulder level with your palms facing up. Stretch your fingers and keep them together. Pull your abdominal muscles in toward your back. Press the small of your back down to the floor. Tighten your buttocks. Relax your neck, toes, shoulders, face, and arms. Press your knees, ankles, and feet together. Then . . .

6b. Breathe out as you sit up straight bringing your arms together in front of you just above shoulder level. Don't slide your feet around or lift them off the floor. Press the palms of your hands together. Keep your elbows straight and your knees, ankles, and feet together. Don't separate your fingers. Stretch each vertebra upward in a straight line. Pull and tighten . . . . Lift your chin slightly. Hold your chest high. Pull your shoulders back and down. Breathe in. Now breathe out as you roll back and down to the position of 6a: Lower your head, aiming your chin to your chest. Gently lay your lower back, waist, rib cage, neck, and then your head on the floor. Open your arms out to the sides.

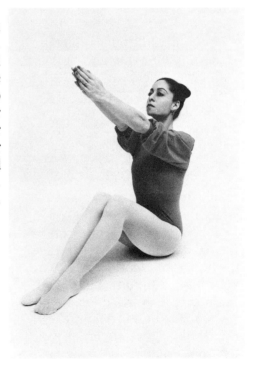

Repeat twice. Remain on your back for exercise #7.

Preparatory Position: *Get Ready!*

On your back with your knees bent and both feet flat on the floor, place your right foot on top of your left knee. Point your right foot. Aim your right knee toward your chin. Rest your arms at your sides. Point your chin toward your chest. Relax your neck, shoulders, face, and left foot. Press the small of your back on the floor. Pull down your abdominal muscles toward your spine. Tighten your buttocks. Let's go!

7a. Breathe in as you raise your arms off the floor and stretch them back to the floor over your head with the palms of your hands facing up. Keep your arms close to your head. Stretch your elbows and fingers. Keep your chin pointed toward your chest. Press the small of your back down to the floor. Remember your abdominal and buttocks muscles. Relax your neck, shoulders, face, and left foot. Then . . .

7b. Breathe out as you raise your arms off the floor and lower them to your sides with the palms of your hands facing down. Don't bend your elbows or move your legs. In one movement, lift your buttocks, pelvis, waist, and rib cage off the floor, aiming both hips upward. Don't arch your back; keep it straight. You should feel as if you're tilting your pelvis up to the ceiling and your rib cage down to the floor. Don't twist your hips or tilt one higher than the other. Be sure to keep your chin inclined toward your chest. Point your right foot. Relax your left foot, shoulders, neck, and face. Pull in and tighten. . . . Now lower your back to the floor gently. Return your arms and body to the position of 7a.

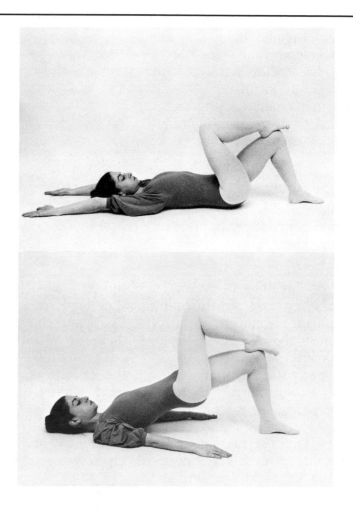

Repeat twice for each leg. Then roll onto your stomach to do exercise #8.

*If you've never exercised before or are very much out of shape, omit this exercise the first week.

Preparatory Position: *Get Ready!*

Lying on your stomach, stretch your legs out together. Bend your elbows and rest your chin on top of your hands. (The palms of your hands are facing down.) Pull in your abdominal muscles. Tighten your buttocks. Point your feet. Relax your neck, fingers, face, and shoulders. Let's go!

8a. Breathe in as you stretch your left arm forward along the floor. Rest your chin on your right hand. Keep your abdominals and buttocks tight, your knees straight, and your feet pointed. Relax your neck, fingers, face, and shoulders. Then . . .

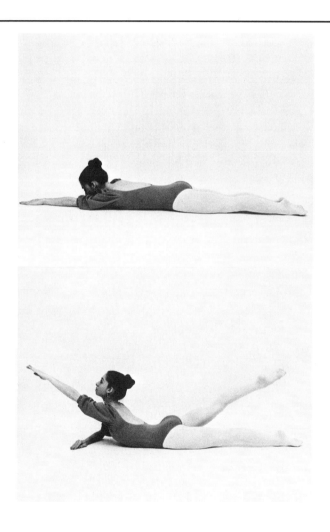

8b. Breathe out as you lift your right leg, left arm, chin, and chest as high off the floor as you can. (Push down into your right forearm and hand for balance and support.) Keep both hips on the floor, especially your right hip. Don't lean to either side. Don't lift your leg or arm out toward either side; keep your body in a straight line. Look over your left hand. Stretch out in opposite directions—from the tips of your fingers to the tips of your toes—to elongate your muscles. Tighten your abdominals and buttocks. Stretch your knees and fingers. Point your feet.

Repeat twice and do the same with your other leg. Then go onto your hands and knees. Place your knees together and your hands shoulder-distance apart. Now turn to exercise #9.

TUESDAY

Preparatory Position: *Get Ready!*

From the starting position, put your right foot, then your left foot, on the floor. Keep your arms straight and your knees and ankles together. Lean into the palms of your hands. Let your heels lift off the floor and your knees bend in between your arms. Pull your abdominals in toward your back. Tighten your buttocks. Let's go!

9a. Breathe in as you shift your weight forward over the palms of your hands. Keep your elbows straight. Lower your head. Try to touch your forehead to your knees. Press your knees and ankles together. Pull in and tighten. Then . . .

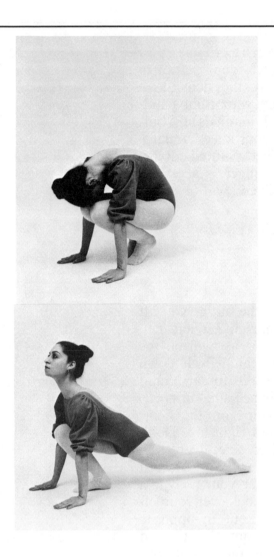

9b. Breathe out as you raise your torso and pelvis and slide your left leg back in alignment with your left shoulder and hip. Point your left foot. Straighten your left knee. Press your right heel to the floor. Keep your right knee in between your arms. Don't bend your elbows or move your hands. Lift your chin and chest upward. Remember your abdominal muscles and buttocks. Stretch your spine long. Don't twist your shoulders—keep them down and back. Push your hips—especially your left one—toward the floor. Finally, bring your left foot back in line with your right foot, the beginning position of 9a.

Repeat twice, alternating legs. Finish in the position of 9a. Then slowly roll through each vertebra to stand up for the next exercise.

TUESDAY

Preparatory Position: *Get Ready!*

Standing erect, put your left foot in front of your right about 12″ apart. Rotate your legs slightly to the outside. Bend your elbows and put your hands on your hips. Then without moving your hips, twist your upper body: bring your right shoulder forward and pull your left shoulder back. Look over your right shoulder. Stretch your spine upward. Pull your abdominal muscles in toward your back and up toward your ribs. Tighten your buttocks. Lift your chest and chin high. Pull your shoulders down. Let's go!

10a. Breathe in as you bend your knees and jump up. Change the position of your legs and shoulders in the air. Bring your right foot in front of your left. Maintain the outward rotation of your legs and their distance of about 12″. Don't move your hands. Twist your upper body. Bring your left shoulder forward and pull your right shoulder back. Keep your shoulders down. Land softly toes to heels. Bend your knees to absorb some of the shock of landing. Don't lift your heels off the floor. Look over your left shoulder. Keep your back straight. Pull in and tighten. Lift your chest and chin high. Then . . .

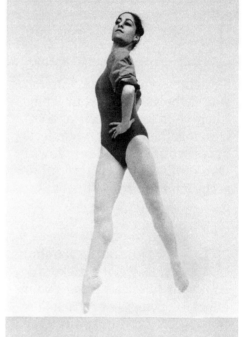

10b. Breathe out as you bend your knees and jump again. This time bring your left foot in front of your right. Continue to rotate your legs to the outside and to maintain a separation of about 12″. Keep your hands on your hips as you twist your upper body, bringing your right shoulder forward and pulling your left shoulder back. Keep your shoulders down. Land softly. Bend your knees. Press your heels on the floor. Look over your right shoulder. Don't let your body sag. Keep your back straight. Remember those abdominal and buttock muscles. Lift your chest and chin high.

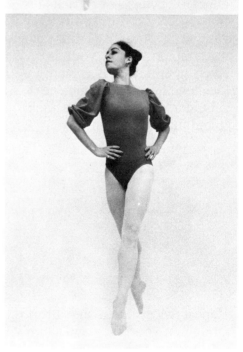

Repeat four times briskly. Now turn to pages 33–34 for the wind-down.

WEDNESDAY

It's important to warm up before any of the sessions. Let's do the exercises in the wind-up section on pages 29–33 and then begin this session.

Preparatory Position: *Get Ready!*

Start on your hands and knees. Put your knees together. Point your fingers forward and place your hands a little wider than shoulder-distance apart and in front of you. Distribute your weight equally between your hands and knees. Pull in your abdominal muscles toward your back. Point your feet. Tighten your buttocks. Let's go!

1a. Breathe in as you shift your weight forward onto the palms of your hands. Straighten your spine. Stretch your elbows. Lift your chin. Keep your knees, feet, and ankles together. Point your feet. Press your shoulders down. Don't tilt your pelvis forward or arch your spine. Pull, tighten. . . . Then . . .

1b. Breathe out as you shift your weight backward. Aim your forehead toward your knees, curving your back forward to stretch your spine. Keep your arms straight. Point your feet. Sit on top of your heels. Keep your knees, feet and ankles together. Relax your neck, shoulders, and face. Remember to pull in and tighten. . . .

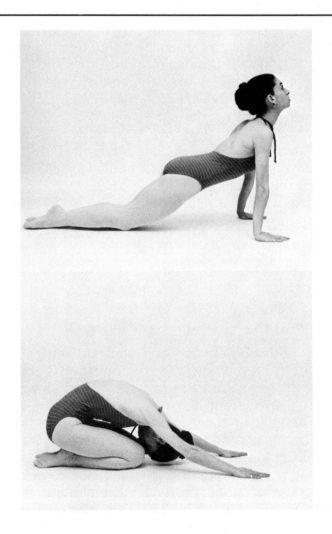

Repeat twice and finish in the position of 1b. Then straighten your back and sit on your heels for the next exercise.

Preparatory Position: *Get Ready!*

As you sit on your heels, keep your knees, feet, and ankles together. (But if you have a special problem, sit as you can.) Point your feet. Don't lean forward or backward. Make sure your hips are in alignment with your shoulders. Pull your weight up off your hips and stretch your spine upward. Now raise your left arm over your head. Flex your left hand back at the wrist, then turn the palm of your hand up and point your fingers to the right. Stretch your fingers and keep them together. Relax your right arm at your side. Hold your chin and chest high. Don't forget to pull in and tighten. Let's go!

2a. Breathe in as you bend to the right side with your left arm straight overhead. Keep your left arm close to your head. Keep your left hand flexed and your fingers pointing right. Extend your right arm out to the side of your body in alignment with your hips. Place the palm of your right hand flat down on the floor with your fingers pointing to the right. Stretch your elbows and fingers. Turn your head and look at your right hand on the floor. Pull in your abdominal muscles toward your back. Tighten your buttocks and don't lift them off your heels. Keep your shoulders back, especially your left one. Keep your chin and chest high. Don't separate your knees, ankles, or feet. Now push off your right hand. Then . . .

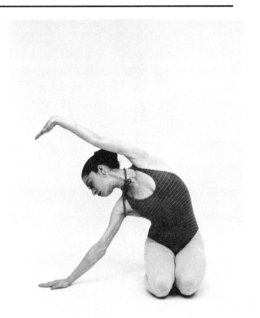

2b. Breathe out as you raise your right arm straight over your head. Flex your right hand back at the wrist and point your fingers to the left. Don't separate your fingers. Keep your right arm close to your head. Bend to the left side. Extend your left arm out to the side of your body in alignment with your hips. Place the palm of your left hand flat down on the floor with your fingers pointing to the left. Stretch your elbows and fingers. Turn your head to the left. Look at your left hand on the floor. Pull in your abdominal muscles toward your back. Tighten your buttocks and keep them on your heels. Keep your shoulders back, especially your right one, and your knees, ankles, and feet together. Hold your chin and chest high. Then push off your left hand to bend to the other side.

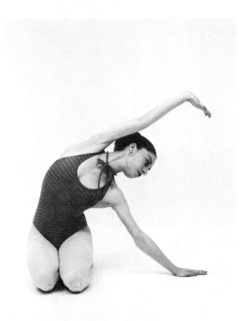

Repeat twice fluidly. Now sit down on your buttocks.

Preparatory Position: *Get Ready!*

Sitting down, bend your knees toward your chest and place your feet lightly on the floor. Keep your knees, feet, and ankles together. Raise your arms over your head. Turn the palms of your hands toward each other. Stretch your spine upward. Abdominal muscles in; buttocks tight. Relax your neck and face. Hold your chin and chest high. Let's go!

3a. Breathe in as you lift your knees toward your chest. Point your feet as they come off the floor. (But if at first it's too difficult to lift your feet off the floor, do this exercise with your toes or feet lightly touching the floor.) Lower your arms to either side at shoulder level. Turn your palms up to the ceiling. Stretch your elbows and fingers. Pull and tighten. Lift your weight up off your hips; feel the space between your hips and ribs. Lengthen each vertebra from the base of your spine up through your neck. Pull your shoulders back and down. Keep your knees, feet, and ankles together. Hold your chin and chest high. Then . . .

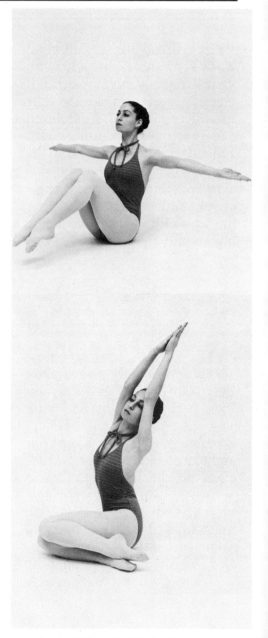

3b. Breathe out as you bring both knees down to the floor on your right side. Draw your feet in close to you. Point your feet. Raise both arms straight over your head close to your ears. Bend to the left side. Don't bend forward at the waist; reach upward through your spine and fingertips. Bend sideways keeping both shoulders back, especially your right one. Keep your chin and chest uplifted. Press the palms of your hands together. Don't separate your fingers. Tilt your head toward your left shoulder. Pull in your abdominals. Tighten your buttocks. Hold your knees, feet, and ankles together.

Repeat four times at a quick pace, alternating sides. Finish in the position of 3b with your left leg on top. Then, go on to exercise #4.

WEDNESDAY

Preparatory Position: *Get Ready!*

Sitting on your right side, place the fingertips of your right hand on the floor about 12″ in front of your right hip. Pull your shoulders back and down, especially your right one. Pull your abdominal muscles in toward your back and up toward your ribs. Lift your weight up off your hips. Hold your chin and chest high. Tighten your buttocks. Look forward. Press your knees, ankles, and inner thighs together. Point your feet. Relax your left arm at your side. Let's go!

4a. Breathe in as you move your left knee forward just past your right knee. Bring your left arm back behind you at shoulder level with the palm of your hand facing down. Position your fingers gracefully. Stretch your spine straight and long. Keep your chin and chest uplifted. Pull your shoulders back and down, especially your right one. Point your feet. Pull and tighten.

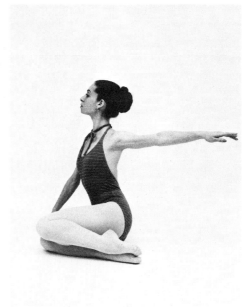

4b. Breathe out as you stretch your left leg back directly behind your left shoulder and hip without touching the floor. Resist rocking your body forward. Continue to stretch your spine. Raise your left arm close to your ear with the palm of your hand facing forward. Don't twist your shoulders. Pull them back and down, especially your right one. Hold your chin and chest high. Remember your abdominal muscles and buttocks. Keep your feet pointed.

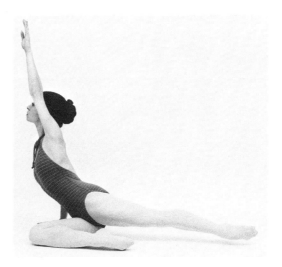

Repeat twice with either leg. Then lie on your back for the next exercise.

★If you've never exercised before or are very much out of shape, omit this exercise the first week.

WEDNESDAY

Preparatory Position: *Get Ready!*

While you're lying on your back, put your legs together. Rest your arms at your sides with the palms of your hands on the floor. Pull your abdominal muscles in toward your back and push the small of your back down to the floor. Bend your left knee to the outside and place your left foot across your right knee. Point your feet. Tighten your buttocks. Relax your face, neck, and shoulders. (If at first 5b is too difficult for you to do, point your chin toward your chest and lift only your head, neck, and upper back off the floor as your arms go forward.) Let's go!

5a. Breathe in as you raise your arms over your head close to your ears with the palms of your hands facing up. Stretch your fingers and keep them together. Pull your abdominals in tight and the small of your back down to the floor. Tighten your buttocks. Keep your right leg and both elbows straight, your left knee bent to the outside, and your feet pointed. Press the outside of your left knee toward the floor without tilting your right hip up. Resist the weight of your left knee and keep both hips on the floor. Stretch your whole body long from the tips of your toes to the tips of your fingers. Then . . .

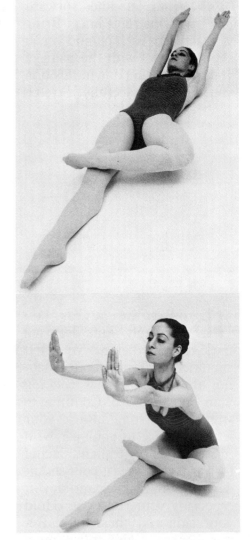

5b. Breathe out as you bring your arms forward to shoulder level and sit up straight. Don't change the position of your legs. Flex your hands back at the wrists. Don't separate your fingers. Lean forward over your legs. Keep your arms and back straight. Point your feet. Lift your chin and look past your fingers. Hold your chest high. Pull in your abdominal muscles. Tighten your buttocks. Stretch your spine long. Keep pressing the outside of your left knee toward the floor without twisting your hips. Now roll back down to the floor. Keep your arms raised and your abdominals and buttocks tight. Don't move your legs. Aim your chin to your chest. Lower your hips, then your waist, rib cage, neck, and head back down to the floor.

Repeat this exercise twice using both legs. Then stand up slowly. For exercise #6 put your heels together, aiming your right foot to the right side and your left foot to the left side. Now bend your knees to the outside. Place the palms of your hands flat on the floor in front of your feet, pointing your fingers toward each other. Pull your abdominals in toward your back and tighten your buttocks.

Preparatory Position: *Get Ready!*

In this squatting position, lean forward onto the palms of your hands. Stretch your elbows and look straight ahead. Turn your heels—which should be off the floor—to the inside so that they face each other. Pull your abdominal muscles in toward your back. Stretch each vertebra upward. Tighten your buttocks. Let's go!

6a. Breathe in as you bend your elbows to the outside. Bend forward, aiming the top of your head at the floor. Pull and tighten. Relax your shoulders, face, and neck. Then . . .

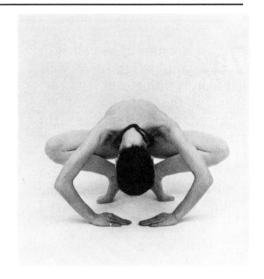

6b. Breathe out as you straighten your elbows and back. Lift your chest and chin as high as you can. Pull your shoulders back and down. Turn your head to the right. Straighten your right leg out to the side, maintaining the outward rotation of your legs and feet. (But if this is too difficult for you, stretch your leg more toward the front and/or bend your knee.) Point your right foot. Shift your weight toward the right and press your left heel on the floor. Don't move your hands or lean backward. Keep your weight inclined forward onto the palms of your hands. Pull your abdominals in toward your back and up toward your ribs. Tighten your buttocks. Stretch your spine straight. Now bend your right knee and slide your right foot along the floor to return to the position of 6a.

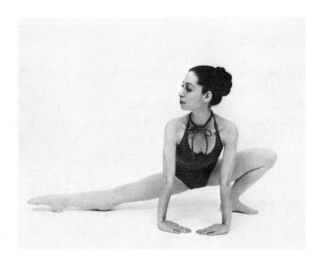

Repeat twice on each side and finish in the position of 6a. Then bring your knees together and stand up slowly to do exercise #7.

Preparatory Position: *Get Ready!*

Stand with your feet placed a little wider than shoulder-distance apart. Turn your feet slightly to the outside and maintain this position throughout this exercise. Distribute your weight equally between your feet, but be light on your heels. Pull up out of your torso and off your hips; stretch each vertebra. Pull and tighten. Now raise your arms above your head a little wider than shoulder-distance apart. Flex your hands back at the wrists. Turn the palms of your hands up, then point your fingertips toward each other. Stretch your elbows. Pull your shoulders back and down. Hold your chin and chest high. Relax your neck. Let's go!

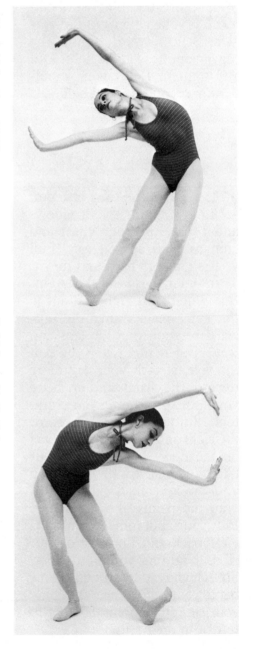

7a. Breathe in as you shift your weight onto your left foot, bending your left knee. Bend at the waist toward the right side and stretch your right knee. Flex your right foot back at the ankle so your right heel is on the floor and your toes are pointed up at an angle to the right. Tilt your head toward your right shoulder. Don't twist your shoulders. Pull them back, especially your left one. Don't let your body sag. Pull your weight up out of your hips. Hold your chin and chest high. Tighten your abdominals and buttocks. Keep your elbows and fingers stretched. Then . . .

7b. Breathe out as you shift your weight onto your right foot. Don't lift your left foot off the floor. Bend your right knee. Bend at the waist to the left side. Don't lean forward or backward. Keep your back straight. Stretch your left knee. Flex your left foot back at the ankle so your left heel is on the floor and your toes are pointing up. Tilt your head toward your left shoulder. Pull both shoulders back, especially your right one. Tighten your abdominals and buttocks. Hold your chin and chest high. Don't bend your elbows or separate your fingers.

Repeat twice smoothly and briskly. Remain standing to do the next exercise.

Preparatory Position: *Get Ready!*

Stand straight with your feet together. Distribute your weight equally on all toes and be light on your heels. Pull your inner thighs toward each other. Stretch your spine long. Lift your weight up off your hips to increase the space between your hips and ribs. Pull your abdominal muscles in toward your back and up toward your ribs. Tighten your buttocks. Relax your neck and toes. Pull your shoulders back and down. Hold your chin and chest high. Now raise your arms above your head a little wider than shoulder-distance apart. Turn the palms of your hands to the outside. Let's go!

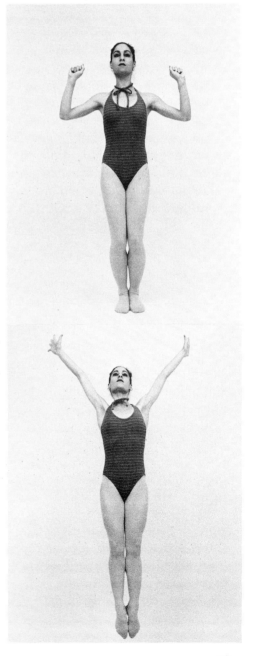

8a. Breathe in as you bend your knees, keeping them together. Press your heels on the floor. Close your hands into tight fists and face them forward. Bend your elbows to the sides and lower them just past shoulder level. Don't lean forward or backward. Align your hips with your shoulders in a perpendicular line. Hold your chin and chest high. Pull and tighten. Then . . .

8b. Breathe out as you jump straight up. Point your feet. Stretch your knees. Keep your back straight, your chin and chest high, and your legs together. Tighten your abdominals and buttocks. Stretch your arms above your head a little wider than shoulder-dis- tance apart. Spread your fingers and turn the palms of your hands to the outside. Then land softly. Roll down through your feet, toes to heels. Keep your knees together as you bend. Pull them in your abdominals and tighten your buttocks.

Repeat four times at a fast pace. Now lie down on your left side to do exercise #9.

Preparatory Position: *Get Ready!*

Lying on your left side, stretch your left arm along the floor past your head with the palm of your hand facing down. Stretch your fingers. Put your right hand on the floor in front of your chest and keep your head up. Point your feet. Make a straight line with your body: align your shoulders, hips, legs, and left arm. Now bend your knees without moving your thighs out of alignment. Slide your lower legs—calves to toes—in toward your buttocks. Don't arch your back. Pull your abdominal muscles in toward your back and up toward your ribs. Tighten your buttocks. Relax your neck. (If at first you have unusual trouble balancing with your body in a straight line, bring your knees and supporting arm further forward.) Let's go!

9a. Breathe in as you raise your right arm and place the palm of your right hand on top of your left hand. Lower your head onto your left arm. Don't move your legs. Press your knees, ankles, and inner thighs together. Pull in your abdominals and tighten your buttocks. Don't twist your shoulders. Pull them back, especially your right one. Keep your feet pointed and back straight. Relax your neck, face, and shoulders. Then . . .

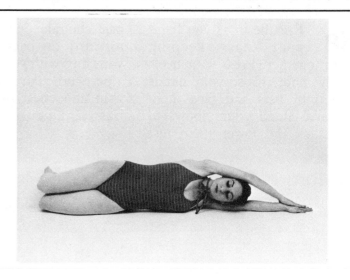

9b. Breathe out as you raise your right arm up and position it at an angle above the right side of your body with the palm of your hand facing down. Position your fingers gracefully. Don't move your left arm. Lift your head up by pushing down onto your left arm. Turn your head to the right and look at your right hand. Raise your right leg up without changing the position of your legs. Keep your shoulders back and down, especially your right one. Point your feet. Pull in and tighten.

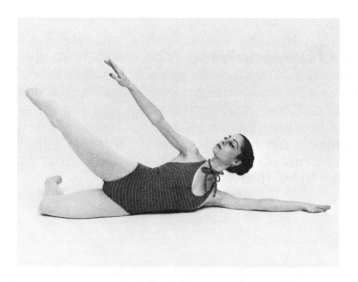

Repeat twice on each side, then roll onto your stomach for the last exercise of this session.

Preparatory Position: *Get Ready!*

Lying on your stomach, stretch your arms straight forward. Interlace your fingers, then turn the palms of your hands away from you. Cross your left ankle on top of your right. Point your feet. Lift your chin, chest, arms, and legs off the floor. Pull in your abdominal muscles toward your back. Tighten your buttocks. Let's go!

10a. Breathe in as you bend your elbows and pull your hands in toward your head. Lower your chest and chin to the floor, but not your elbows. Keep your fingers interlaced and the palms of your hands facing out. Pushing your left ankle against your right, bend your knees. Aim your feet toward your buttocks. Keep your knees together, your hips on the floor, and your feet pointed. Tighten your abdominals and buttocks. Then . . .

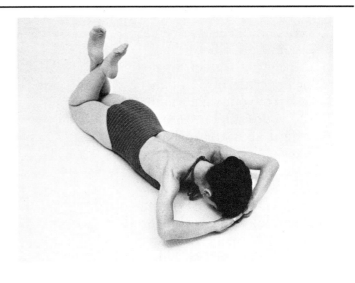

10b. Breathe out as you straighten your elbows, lifting your chin, chest, and arms up. Don't separate your hands. Pushing your left ankle against your right, straighten your knees and raise your legs off the floor. Keep your legs together and your feet pointed. Pull in and tighten.

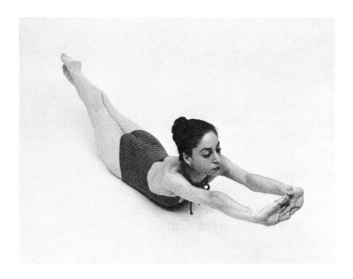

Repeat twice, then do the same exercise with your right ankle crossed on top of your left one. Stand up slowly. Now you're ready to do the wind-down. Turn to pages 33–34 and follow me.

THURSDAY

Have you done the wind-up exercises yet? If not, turn to pages 29–33 and follow them. Then you'll be ready to start today's session.

Preparatory Position: *Get Ready!*

Lie down on your left side. Align your left elbow underneath your left shoulder and lean on it. Place the palm of your left hand flat on the floor at a right angle to your body. Put your legs together. Point your feet. Pull in your abdominal muscles toward your back. Tighten your buttocks. Hold your chin and chest high. Now raise your right arm out to the side above shoulder level with the palm of your hand facing up. Stretch your fingers and keep them together. Make sure your body is properly aligned: your legs, hips, shoulders, and right arm should all be in the same plane. Let's go!

1a. Breathe in as you bend your right elbow. Don't drop it below shoulder level. Place the fingertips of your right hand on top of your right shoulder. Bend your right knee lifting it up toward your right elbow. Keep your left leg straight. Turn your head to the left side and look past your left hand. Point your feet. Don't twist your shoulders. Pull them back and down, especially your left one. Don't sink onto your left side. Push down onto your left forearm and hand to lift the left side of your body off the floor. Pull in and tighten. Hold your chin and chest high. Keep your back straight. Then . . .

1b. Breathe out as you straighten your right elbow, stretching your right arm to the side above shoulder level. Turn the palm of your hand up. Don't separate your fingers. Straighten your right leg, lifting it as close to your right arm as possible. Don't move either leg forward or backward. Keep them in a plane with your hips, shoulders, and right arm. Turn your head to the right and look past your right hand. Keep your feet pointed. Hold your chin and chest high. Pull your shoulders back and down, especially your left one. Pull in and tighten. Push down onto your left forearm and hand to keep the left side of your body elevated.

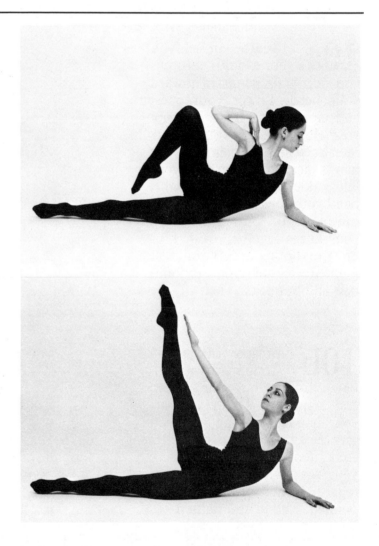

Repeat twice on your left side and twice on your right. Then roll onto your stomach to do the next exercise.

Preparatory Position: *Get Ready!*

Lying on your stomach, separate your legs and extend your arms forward with the palms of your hands facing down. Stretch your fingers and keep them together. Point your feet. Lift your legs, chest, and arms off the floor. Pull your abdominal muscles in toward your back and tighten your buttocks. Pull your shoulders back and down. Relax your neck and face. Let's go!

2a. Breathe in as you bring your legs together, lowering them slightly toward the floor. You should feel great resistance as if you are pushing against a wall of bricks. With your arms off the floor, bring them from front to back, turning the palms of your hands up.

Keep your fingers together. Lower your head and chest toward the floor. Stretch your elbows, fingers, and knees. Point your feet. Pull in your abdominal muscles. Tighten your buttocks. Stretch your back from the base of your spine up through your neck. Then . . .

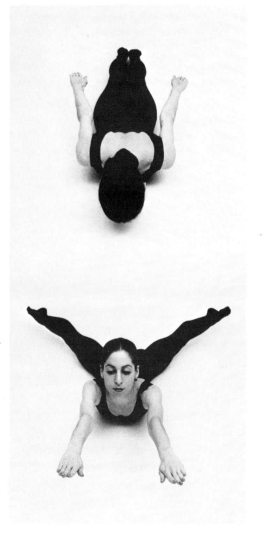

2b. Breathe out as you pull your legs apart—again, feeling the resistance—lifting them as high as you can. Keeping your arms off the floor, bring them from back to front, turning the palms of your hands down.

Keep your fingers together. Raise your chin and chest up off the floor. Pull your shoulders back and down. Stretch your elbows, knees, and fingers. Point your feet. Pull in and tighten.

Repeat twice slowly. Then, go onto your hands and knees for exercise #3!

Preparatory Position: *Get Ready!*

Put your knees together and place one hand on top of the other. Bend your elbows and lower them onto the floor. Rest your forehead on top of your hands. Relax your neck and face. Slide your right foot back directly behind your right hip and shoulder, stretching your right knee. Then lift your right leg off the floor as high as you can. Stretch your spine straight. Pull your shoulders down and back by pushing down onto your elbows, forearms, and hands. Pull in your abdominal muscles toward your back and tighten your buttocks. Point your feet. Don't lean toward either side; distribute your weight equally between your elbows, hands, and left knee. Let's go!

3a. Breathe in as you bend your right knee smoothly without lowering your leg or changing its direction. Flex your right foot back at the ankle, aiming the sole of your foot toward the ceiling. Point your left foot. Don't cave in at the waist. Keep your back straight and your shoulders and hips even. Pull in and tighten. Pull your shoulders back and down. Relax your neck and face. Then . . .

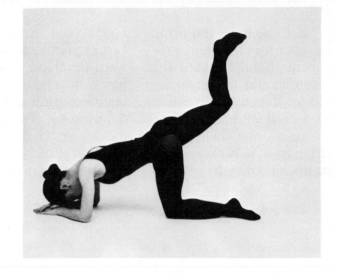

3b. Breathe out as you straighten your right knee smoothly without lowering your leg. Don't let your leg drift out toward the side. Point your right foot. Aim the back of your right leg and the sole of your foot toward the ceiling. Don't twist your shoulders or hips. Keep your back straight, abdominals pulled in, buttocks tight, shoulders back and down, neck and face relaxed, and left foot pointed.

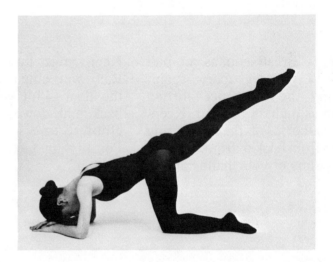

Repeat twice with each leg. Then stand up slowly. Turn to exercise #4.

THURSDAY

Preparatory Position: *Get Ready!*

Stand with your feet a little wider than shoulder-distance apart and point your feet forward. Pull your abdominal muscles in toward your spine and up toward your ribs. Tighten your buttocks. Stretch your back to increase the distance between your hips and ribs. Distribute your weight equally on your legs but lean slightly forward over your toes. Be light on your heels. Open your arms out to the sides at shoulder level with the palms of your hands facing forward. Position your fingers gracefully. Relax your neck and toes. Hold your chest and chin high. Let's go!

4a. Breathe in as you bend your knees. Don't lift your heels off the floor. Raise your left arm over your head in a gentle curve with the palm of your hand facing the middle of your head. Curve your right arm in front of your legs, turning the palm of your hand up. Bend at the waist to the right side. Keep your back straight. Don't bend forward or backward. Turn your head to the right and look over your right shoulder. Pull in your abdominal muscles. Tighten your buttocks. Pull your shoulders back and down, especially your left one. Hold your chin and chest high. Then . . .

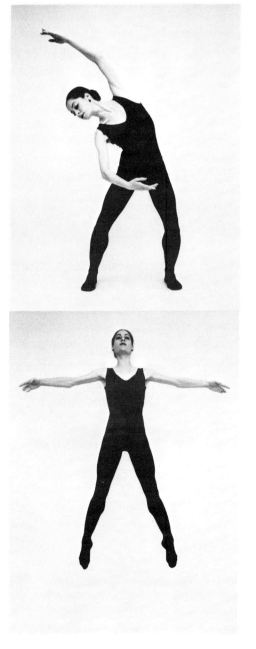

4b. Breathe out as you stand up again, stretching your back. Look forward. Stretch both arms out to the sides at shoulder level. Turn the palms of your hands forward. Then jump up. Stretch your knees. Point your feet. Don't let your legs "wander" when you jump. Land softly, raising your right arm in a graceful curve above your head and lowering your left curved in front of your legs. Bend your torso to the left but keep your back straight. Hold your chin and chest high. Remember your abdominal muscles and buttocks. Pull your weight up off your hips. Don't twist your shoulders. Pull them back and down, especially your right one. Now return to 4a: Breathe in. Jump (4b). Breathe out, landing softly into the position of 4a.

Repeat four times vigorously. Remain standing for exercise #5.

THURSDAY

Preparatory Position: *Get Ready!*

Standing erect, put your legs together with your heels touching and toes pointing slightly to the outside. Stretch your spine. Pull your abdominal muscles in toward your back and up toward your ribs. Tighten your buttocks. Pull your weight up off your hips. Hold your chest and chin high. Relax your toes and neck. Pull your shoulders down and back. Now slide your left leg back diagonally, crossing your legs at the tops of your thighs and stretching up on the ball of your left foot. Distribute your weight equally on both legs. Raise your arms over your head next to your ears. Press the palms of your hands together. Relax your elbows. Turn your head to the right. Don't arch your back. Try tilting your pelvis slightly forward to keep your back straight. Let's go!

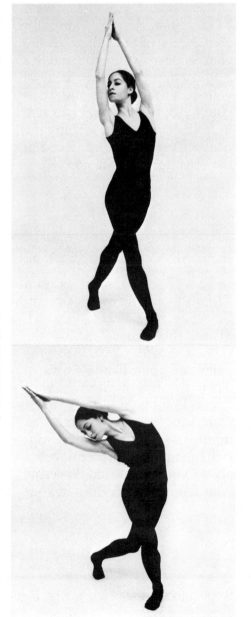

5a. Breathe in as you stretch your whole body upward. Align your hips, shoulders, and hands. Pull in your abdominal muscles and tighten your buttocks. Stretch your knees. Don't twist your shoulders. Pull them back and down. Relax the toes of your right foot. Keep your head turned to the right, your weight equally distributed between your front and back legs, the palms of your hands pressed together and your arms raised next to your ears. Hold your chin and chest high. Then . . .

5b. Breathe out as you bend your knees. Don't lift your right heel off the floor. Bend at the waist to the right side. Don't bend forward, arch your spine backward, separate your hands, or lower your arms. Pull your shoulders back and down, especially your left one. Hold your chest and chin high. Abdominal muscles in and buttocks tight! Keep your head turned to the right and your back straight.

Repeat twice on either side. Remain standing! Exercise #6 is next.

THURSDAY

Preparatory Position: *Get Ready!*

Stand erect with your feet a bit wider than shoulder-distance apart. Turn your legs slightly toward the outside. Bend forward from your hips—not from your waist—stretching your spine straight. Your arms in front of your shoulders, point your fingers toward each other and press the palms of your hands on the floor. Stretch your elbows. (But if at first you do not have enough flexibility to do this exercise as it is, don't worry about pressing the palms of your hands on the floor or straightening your knees and elbows.) Distribute your weight equally between your hands and feet. Pull your abdominal muscles up toward your back. Tighten your buttocks. Let's go!

6a. Breathe in as you bend your knees toward the outside. Don't lift your heels off the floor. Keep your back straight. Lower your chest, waist, and hips toward the floor but raise your buttocks, chin, and chest upward. Pull in and tighten. Pull your shoulders down and back. Then . . .

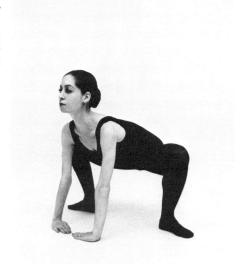

6b. Breathe out as you straighten and stretch your knees. Keep your elbows straight. Don't move your hands or feet. Do not turn your legs to the inside. Roll onto your heels, lifting your toes off the floor. Lower your chin toward your chest. Look through your legs. Pull in and tighten. Distribute your weight equally between your heels and hands.

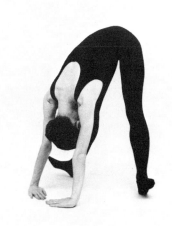

Repeat twice. Then sit down. Turn to exercise #7.

Preparatory Position: *Get Ready!*

While in a sitting position, put your legs together. Point your fingers out to the sides and place the palms of your hands on the floor behind you, a little wider than shoulder-distance apart. Pull your abdominal muscles in toward your back and up toward your ribs. Stretch each vertebra from the base of your spine through the middle of your head. Pull your weight up off your hips. Pull your shoulders back and down. Hold your chin and chest high. Tighten your buttocks. Point your feet. Now lean back into the palms of your hands without caving in at the waist. Let's go!

7a. Breathe in as you shift your weight onto the palm of your right hand. Your fingers should still be pointing to the right side. Bend your right elbow slightly. Don't let it touch the floor. Roll onto the right side of your buttocks, hips, and legs. Point your feet. Slide the inside of your left ankle up along your right leg to the top of your inner thigh aiming your left knee at the floor. Don't bend your right knee. Raise your left arm to the side just above shoulder level with the palm of your hand facing down. Position your fingers gracefully. Turn your head to the left and look past your left hand. Pull your shoulders down and back. Keep your back straight, chin and chest lifted, abdominals pulled in and buttocks tight. Then push off your right hand. Put your left hand on the floor, pointing your fingers to the left side. Slide the inside of your left ankle down along the inside of your right leg. Stretch your left leg. Then . . .

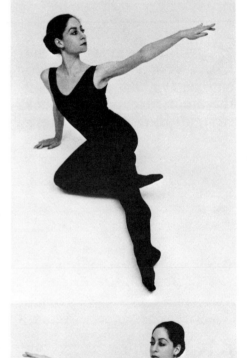

7b. Breathe out as you shift your weight onto the palm of your left hand. Bend your left elbow slightly but don't let it touch the floor. Roll onto the left side of your buttocks, hips, and legs. Point your feet. Slide the inside of your right ankle up along your left leg to the top of your inner thigh. Aim your right knee at the floor. Keep your left leg straight. Raise your right arm to a point just above shoulder level on your right side, the palm of your hand facing down. Position your fingers gracefully. Turn your head to the right and look past your right hand. Pull your shoulders back and down. Keep your back straight, pull your abdominal muscles in and tighten your buttocks. Hold your chin and chest high. Now push off your left hand. Put your right hand on the floor, pointing your fingers to the right side. Slide the inside of your right ankle down along the inside of your left leg and stretch through your toes.

Repeat four times at a brisk pace. Then lie down on your back to do exercise #8.

THURSDAY

Preparatory Position: *Get Ready!*

Lying on your back, bend your knees toward your chest. Put your knees and ankles together. Rest your arms at your sides with the palms of your hands facing down. Relax your neck, face, and shoulders. Press the small of your back down to the floor. Pull your abdominal muscles down toward your back. Tighten your buttocks. Let's go!

8a. Breathe in as you pull your knees as close to your chest as you can with your buttocks on the floor. Don't move your arms. Point your chin toward your chest. Pull in and tighten. Point your feet. Relax your neck, face, and shoulders. Then . . .

8b. Breathe out as you bring your knees above your head toward the floor. Keep your knees and ankles together. Place your hands behind your waist to support your back. And don't let go! Press your chin toward your chest. Relax your neck, face, and shoulders. Straighten your knees. Don't separate your legs. Try to touch the floor with your feet. (If this is too difficult for you to do at this time, bring your knees toward your head or if you can, above your head, but don't straighten them or touch the floor with your feet. Support your back with your hands and uncoil as instructed.) Pull your abdominal muscles in and tighten your buttocks. Keep holding on to your back! Take a deep breath. Then breathe out very slowly as you bend your knees. Slide your hands up toward your buttocks to help you control your de-

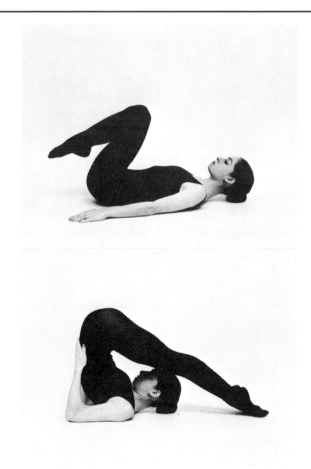

scent. Keep your chin pointed toward your chest. Relax your neck, face, and shoulders. Don't drop or kick your legs. Gradually lower each vertebra to the floor and finish in the position of 8a.

Do not repeat. Stay in the position of 8a for exercise #9.

*If you've never exercised before or are very much out of shape, omit this exercise the first week.

73

Preparatory Position: *Get Ready!*

From the position of 8a, raise your feet higher than your knees. Raise your arms in front of your shoulders, above the level of your knees. Turn the palms of your hands down. Keep your knees and ankles together, feet pointed and the small of your back on the floor. Pull your abdominal muscles down toward your back. Tighten your buttocks. Let's go!

9a. Breathe in as you flex your feet back at the ankles. Rest your head on the floor. Relax your shoulders, face, and neck. Stretch your elbows. Keep your arms forward in front of your shoulders with the palms of your hands facing down. Don't let them drop! Stretch your fingers and hold them together. Pull . . . tighten . . . and press the small of your back down to the floor. Then . . .

9b. Breathe out as you point your chin toward your chest. Point your feet. Lift your upper back off the floor. Don't change the height of your arms, bring your knees down toward your chest, or drop your feet lower than your knees. Reach past your knees with the palms of your hands facing down. Don't separate your fingers. Keep your elbows straight and your knees and ankles together. Pull your abdominals down toward your back. Tighten your buttocks and don't let them off the floor. Return to the position of 9a. Keep your arms raised and your chin inclined toward your chest.

Repeat twice. Stay on your back for the next exercise.

THURSDAY

x

THURSDAY

stop

THURSDAY   #10

Preparatory Position: *Get Ready!*

Lying on your back, bend your knees and place your feet flat on the floor. Put your knees, ankles, and feet together. Pull your abdominal muscles down toward your back and up toward your ribs. Press the small of your back down to the floor.

Tighten your buttocks. Interlace your fingers, then turn the palms of your hands out. Stretch your arms past your head, in alignment with the rest of your body. Relax your neck, face, toes, and shoulders. Let's go!

10a. Breathe in as you lower your arms below shoulder level. Keep your elbows straight, your fingers interlaced, and your knees, ankles, and feet together. Push upward through the palms of your hands. Pull in your abdominals and tighten your buttocks. Relax your neck, face, shoulders, and toes. Press the small of your back down to the floor. Then . . .

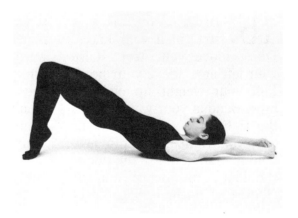

10b. Breathe out as you lower your arms past your head with the palms of your hands facing out. Don't bend your elbows or separate your fingers. Raise your buttocks, pelvis, waist, and rib cage off the floor in one movement. Point your chin toward your chest. Keep your knees, ankles, and feet together. Rise onto the balls of your feet, lifting your heels off the floor as much as you can. Don't arch your back. It's helpful to tilt your pelvis up to the ceiling and your rib cage down to the floor to help you keep your back straight. Don't twist your hips. Keep them parallel to the ceiling. Relax your neck, face, and shoulders. Stretch your whole body from your hands to your toes. Now gently lower your back, heels, and arms into the position of 10a.

Repeat twice. Roll onto your right side. Put both feet on the floor, then stand up slowly. Turn to pages 33–34. Let's do the wind-down.

75

FRIDAY

Before you start this session, warm up with the exercises pictured and described in the wind-up section, pages 29–33.

Preparatory Position: *Get Ready!*

Stand erect with your feet placed a little wider than shoulder-distance apart. Turn your legs slightly to the outside and distribute your weight equally on both legs. Stretch your arms out to the sides at shoulder level. Turn the palms of your hands up. Pull your abdominal muscles in toward your back and up toward your ribs. Tighten your buttocks. Stretch each vertebra and pull your weight up out of your torso. Hold your chin and chest high. Pull your shoulders down and back. Relax your neck and toes. Let's go!

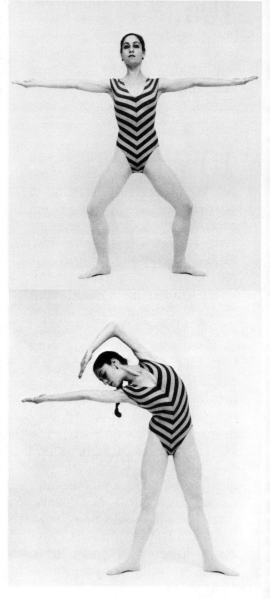

1a. Breathe in as you bend your knees to the outside. Don't lift your heels off the floor. Straighten your elbows and hold your arms out to the sides at shoulder level with the palms of your hands facing up. Stretch your fingers and keep them together. Look straight ahead. Stretch your spine upward. Pull your shoulders down and back. Hold your chin and chest high. Pull in your abdominals. Tighten your buttocks. Then . . .

1b. Breathe out as you straighten your knees. Don't move your feet. Raise your left arm above your head. Pull your weight up off your hips. Bend at your waist toward the right side. Don't bend or drop your right arm; continue to hold it straight out to the side at shoulder level. Bend your left elbow toward the ceiling. Don't separate your fingers. Aim the fingertips of your left hand toward the middle of your right arm. Turn your head to the right and look at your right arm. Don't twist your shoulders. Pull them back and down, especially your left one. Pull in and tighten. Hold your chin and chest high.

Repeat twice fluidly, alternating sides. Remain standing for exercise #2.

Preparatory Position: *Get Ready!*

Stand with your feet placed more than shoulder-distance apart and your legs and feet rotated slightly toward the outside. Turn your left foot forward. Now bend forward toward your right leg and place the palms of your hands on the floor to either side of your right foot. (But if at first this is too difficult, try to touch the floor with your fingertips or whatever you can do until you have the required flexibility.) Pull your abdominal muscles in toward your back. Relax your shoulders, face, and neck. Tighten your buttocks. Let's go!

2a. Breathe in as you shift your weight backward onto your left foot. Don't move your hands. Bend your left knee, then stretch your right. Flex your right foot back at the ankle, lifting your toes off the floor. Keep your left heel on the floor and your elbows and fingers straight. Lift your chin and chest upward. Pull in your abdominal muscles. Tighten your buttocks and aim them upward. Stretch your spine long. Pull your shoulders down and back. Then . . .

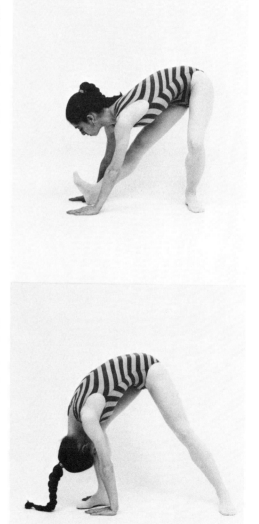

2b. Breathe out as you shift your weight forward onto your right foot, returning your right toes to the floor. Don't move your hands. Bend your right knee as you stretch your left knee. But keep both heels on the floor! Lower your head, aiming your forehead at your right knee. Pull in your abdominal muscles. Tighten your buttocks and aim them downward. Don't bend your elbows. Relax your face, toes, neck, and shoulders.

Repeat twice, stretching toward either side. Stand up slowly for the next exercise.

FRIDAY

Preparatory Position: *Get Ready!*

Stand erect. Place your feet a little wider than shoulder-distance apart with your feet facing forward. Pull your weight up off your hips and stretch your spine upward. Be light on your heels. Pull your abdominal muscles in toward your back and up toward your ribs. Tighten your buttocks. Hold your chin and chest high. Pull your shoulders back and down. Stretch your arms out to the sides at shoulder level, with the palms of your hands facing back. Spread your fingers apart. Now bend forward from your hips keeping your back straight and your chin and chest raised. Look straight ahead. Let's go!

3a. Breathe in as you shift your weight onto your right foot. Bend your right knee. Swing your left arm down diagonally across toward the right side. Raise your right arm up slightly past shoulder level. Don't bend your elbows. Spread your fingers apart and turn the palms of your hands back. Turn your head toward the right side and look up at your right hand. Straighten your left knee. Flex your left foot back at the ankle, lifting the toes of your left foot off the floor. But don't lean backward, you'll throw yourself off balance. Pull your shoulders down and back. Tighten your abdominal and buttock muscles. Keep your back straight and your chin and chest raised. Then . . .

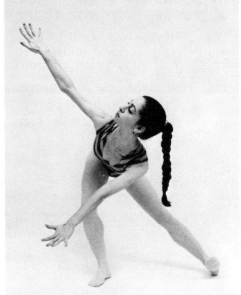

3b. Breathe out as you shift your weight onto your left foot, putting your toes on the floor. Bend your left knee. Swing your right arm down diagonally toward the left side. Raise your left arm to the side, slightly past shoulder level. Don't bend your elbows. Continue to spread your fingers and turn the palms of your hands back. Turn your head toward the left side and look up at your left hand. Straighten your right knee. Flex your right foot back at the ankle, lifting your toes off the floor. Don't lean backward. Pull your shoulders down and back. Pull in and tighten. Keep your back straight. Aim your buttocks up to the ceiling and hold your chin and chest high.

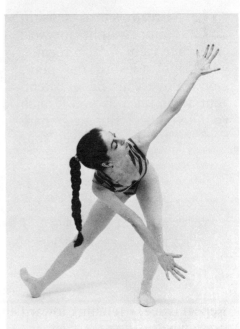

Repeat four times briskly. Then slowly stand upright and go on to exercise #4.

FRIDAY

Preparatory Position: *Get Ready!*

Stand erect. Put your right foot in front of your left about 15″ apart. Turn your legs slightly to the outside. Distribute your weight equally on both legs. Pull your abdominal muscles in toward your back and up toward your ribs. Stretch your spine upward. Hold your chin and chest high. Pull your shoulders back and down. Tighten your buttocks. Let's go!

4a. Breathe in as you bend your knees. Don't lift your heels off the floor. Bend your elbows toward the outside and press the palms of your hands together in front of your chest. Turn your head toward your left shoulder and look down at your left knee. Twist your upper body toward the left. Tighten your abdominals and buttocks. Hold your chin and chest high. Keep your shoulders down and your back straight.

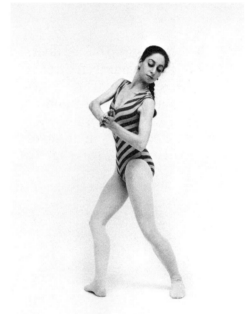

4b. Now jump off the floor. Point your feet. Stretch your knees. Separate your hands. Change the direction of your body as you bring your left leg in front of your right about 15″ apart. Rotate your legs slightly to the outside. Keep your back straight. Remember your abdominal muscles and buttocks. Hold your chin and chest high. Pull your shoulders down. Then . . .

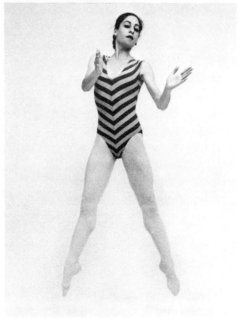

4c. Breathe out as you land, rolling from the balls of your feet to your heels and bending your knees. Press your heels on the floor. Your left foot is about 15″ in front of your right. Distribute your weight equally on both feet. With your elbows bent to the outside, press the palms of your hands together in front of your chest. Turn your head toward your right shoulder and look down at your right knee. Twist your upper body toward the right. Tighten your abdominals and buttocks. Hold your chin and chest high. Pull your shoulders down.

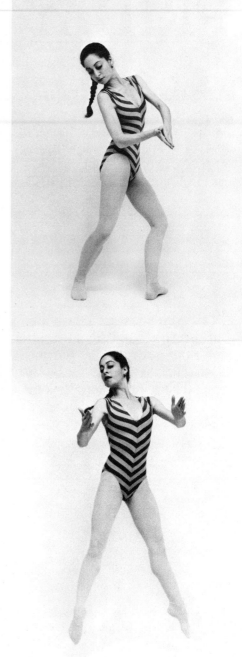

4d. Now jump off the floor. Point your feet. Stretch your knees. Separate your hands. Change the direction of your body as you bring your right leg about 15″ in front of your left. Turn your legs slightly to the outside. Land in the position of 4a. Distribute your weight equally on both feet. Keep your back straight, abdominal muscles and buttocks tight, chest high, and your shoulders back and down.

Repeat twice at a brisk pace. Then lie down on your stomach to be ready for exercise #5.

80

FRIDAY

Preparatory Position: *Get Ready!*

Lying down on your stomach, stretch your legs apart and extend your arms out to the sides at shoulder level, with the palms of your hands facing down. Flex your feet back at the ankles. Pull in your abdominal muscles and tighten your buttocks. Relax your shoulders, face, and neck. Let's go!

5a. Breathe in as you straighten your knees and pull your legs together. Point your feet. Straighten your elbows. The palms of your hands should still be turned down and your arms should be out to your sides, held steady at shoulder level. Rest your chin and chest on the floor. Stretch your spine long. Press your hips down to the floor. Pull in and tighten your abdominal and buttock muscles. Relax your shoulders, neck, and face. Then . . .

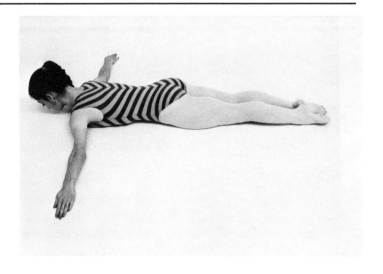

5b. Breathe out as you bend your elbows, sliding your forearms and hands forward. Don't move your elbows. Push down onto your forearms and hands and lift your chin and chest off the floor. Look up. Bend your knees to the outside and slide them up along the floor. Press your heels together and flex your feet back at the ankles. Don't let your hips leave the floor. Don't twist your shoulders. Pull your shoulders back and down. Pull in and tighten.

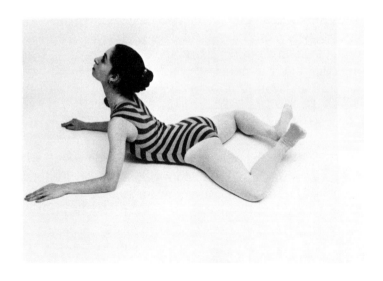

Repeat twice. Roll onto your left side for exercise #6.

*If you've never exercised before or are very much out of shape, omit this exercise the first week.

FRIDAY

Preparatory Position: *Get Ready!*

Lying on your left side, place your left elbow underneath your left shoulder and lean on it. Place the palm of your left hand flat on the floor facing forward. Put the palm of your right hand on the floor a small distance in front of your waist. Stretch your legs straight out to the side and align them with your hips, shoulders, and left elbow. Point your feet. Pull your abdominal muscles in toward your back. Tighten your buttocks. Don't let your left side collapse; push down onto your left forearm and hand to lift it off the floor. Pull your shoulders down and back, especially your left one. Hold your chin and chest high. Now slide your right foot along your left leg, bending your right knee up toward the ceiling. Point your right foot by your left knee. Let's go!

6a. Breathe in as you lower your right knee to the floor, keeping the toes of your right foot by your left knee. Don't bend your left leg. Keep your feet pointed. Raise your right arm to the side at shoulder level with the palm of your hand facing up. Stretch your fingers and keep them together. Turn your head to the right. Look past your right hand. Don't twist your shoulders. Pull them back and down, especially your left one. Pull in your abdominal muscles and tighten your buttocks. Hold your chin and chest high. Don't let your left side collapse! Then . . .

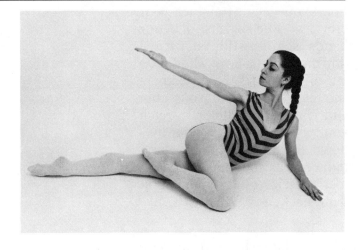

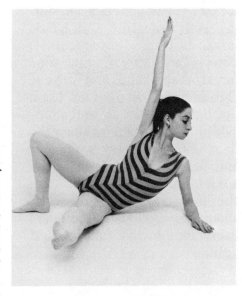

6b. Breathe out as you raise your right arm above your head with the palm of your hand facing left. Don't separate your fingers. Pull your right knee back, aiming your kneecap toward the ceiling. Place your right foot flat on the floor behind your left knee. Raising your left leg off the floor, swing it straight in front of you. Keep your left foot pointed. Turn your head to the left side. Look past your left shoulder. Pull your shoulders back and down, especially your left one. Pull in your abdominal muscles and tighten your buttocks. Hold your chin and chest high. To prevent the left side of your torso from sagging, push down onto your left forearm and hand. To return to 6a, swing your left leg back and place it on the floor in alignment with your shoulders, hips, and left elbow. Point your right foot at the side of your left knee.

Repeat twice on each side. Then lie on your back for the next exercise.

FRIDAY

Preparatory Position: *Get Ready!*

Lying on your back, put your legs together and extend your arms out to the sides at shoulder level with the palms of your hands facing down. Bend your knees slightly, placing your feet flat on the floor. Keep your knees, ankles, and feet together.

Pull your abdominal muscles down toward your back. Tighten your buttocks! Press the small of your back down to the floor. Relax your neck, face, and shoulders. Let's go!

7a. Breathe in as you lower your knees toward the floor on the left side. Don't move your arms or feet, or separate your legs. Keep your shoulders and upper back on the floor. Relax your neck and face. Pull in your abdominal muscles and tighten your buttocks. Point your feet. Then . . .

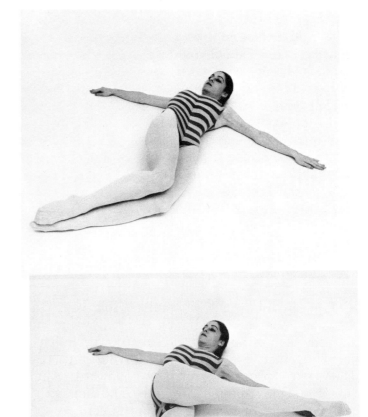

7b. Breathe out as you straighten your right leg, kicking it up toward your left hand. Don't move your arms or your left leg. Keep your shoulders and upper back on the floor and your feet pointed. Relax your neck and face. Pull in and tighten. Then return to the position of 7a by bending your right knee and placing it on top of your left knee.

Repeat twice on each side. Stay on your back to do exercise #8.

FRIDAY

Preparatory Position: *Get Ready!*

Lying on your back, put your legs together flat on the floor and extend your arms out to the sides at shoulder level, with the palms of your hands facing down. Bend your knees slightly and place both feet flat on the floor. Keep your knees, ankles, and feet together. Remember your abdominal muscles and buttocks! Press the small of your back down to the floor. Relax your neck, face, and shoulders. Let's go!

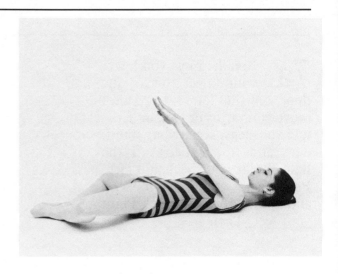

8a. Breathe in as you push your knees and ankles away from each other toward the floor. Press the soles of your feet together. Bring your arms together over your stomach. Stretch your elbows. Turn the palms of your hands toward your hips. Stretch your fingers and keep them together. Pull in your abdominal muscles and tighten your buttocks. Press the small of your back down to the floor. Point your chin toward your chest. Stretch your spine along the floor. Relax your face and neck. Then . . .

8b. Breathe out as you pull your knees and ankles toward each other and press them together. Sit up straight. Don't move your feet. (But if at first this is too strenuous for you to do because of weak back or weak abdominal muscles, don't sit up completely. Lift only your head, neck, and shoulders from the floor instead of your whole back.) Raise your arms above your head at a slightly more open angle. Don't bend your elbows. Turn the palms of your hands out toward the sides. Don't separate your fingers.

Hold your chin and chest high. Pull your shoulders back and down. Pull your weight up off your hips. Stretch your spine upward. Align your shoulders and hips so your shoulders are directly on top of your hips. Tighten your abdominals and buttocks. To return to the position of 8a, lower your head, aiming your chin at your chest. Roll down to the floor through each vertebra, starting from the base of your spine. Tighten your abdominals and buttocks. Lower your arms over your torso.

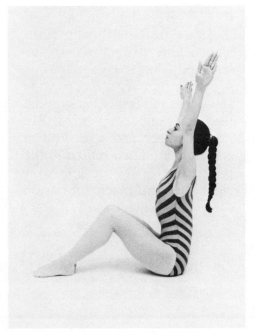

Repeat twice. Finish in the position of 8b. Then go on to exercise #9

FRIDAY

Preparatory Position: *Get Ready!*

Sit as erect as you can, with your legs straight out in front of you. Increase the space between your hips and your ribs by pulling each vertebra upward. Pull in and tighten. Pull your shoulders back and down. Hold your chin and chest high. Extend your arms out to the sides at shoulder level, the palms of your hands facing down. Then flex your hands back at the wrists so that your fingers point up. Stretch your fingers and hold them together. Point your right foot. Flex your left foot back at the ankle. Then, raise your left leg off the floor but keep your back straight. You should be in the 9b position. Let's go!

9a. Breathe in as you bend your left knee toward your left shoulder. Keep your right leg straight. Lean back. Lower your head, aiming your forehead toward your knee cap. Bring your arms forward at shoulder level. Your arms should be straight and your hands flexed back at the wrists. Don't separate your fingers. Pull in your abdominal muscles. Tighten your buttocks. Keep your left foot flexed back at the ankle and your right foot pointed. Then . . .

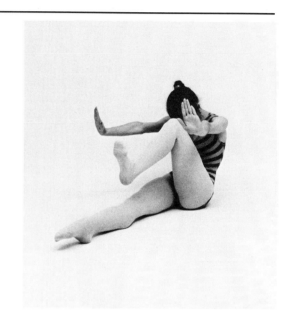

9b. Breathe out as you stretch your spine and sit up straight. Pull your weight up off your hips. Stretch your left knee. Try not to lower your leg. Keep your left foot flexed back at the ankle, your right foot pointed and your right leg straight. Open your arms out to the sides at shoulder level. Keep your hands flexed back at the wrists and your fingers together. Raise your chin and chest upward. Pull your shoulders back and down. Pull in and tighten.

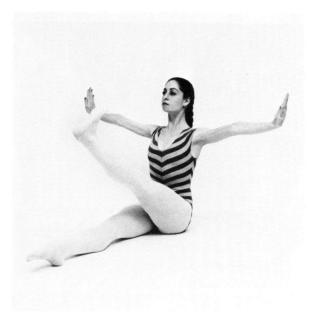

Repeat twice with each leg. Stay seated. Exercise #10 is next!

FRIDAY

Preparatory Position: *Get Ready!*

As you sit with your legs straight out in front of you, bend your knees toward your chest. Keep your knees and feet together. Lower your knees to the floor on the right side. Pull your feet toward your buttocks and point them. Place your fingertips on the floor in front of your hips. Pull both shoulders down and back, especially your right one. Lift your chin and chest high. Pull your abdominal muscles in toward your back and up toward your ribs. Stretch your back long. Don't lean toward the right side. Now lift your left leg and extend it directly back behind your left shoulder and hip. Let's go!

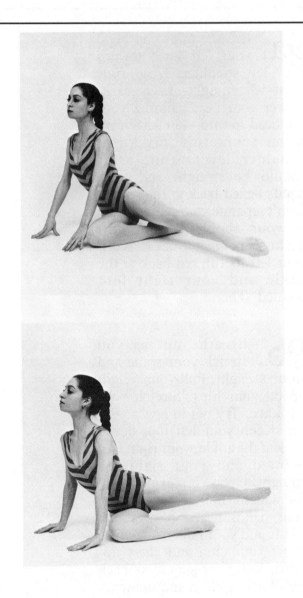

10a. Breathe in as you swing your left leg to the side, keeping it straight and off the floor. Don't move your right leg. Distribute your weight equally between your fingertips. Pull your shoulders back and down, especially your right one. Lift your chin and chest high. Pull in your abdominals and tighten your buttocks. Stretch your back upward. Then . . .

10b. Breathe out as you swing your left leg back directly behind your left shoulder and hip. Don't move your right leg. Don't bend your left leg or drop it to the floor. Press the palms of your hands down on the floor. Straighten your elbows. Don't twist your shoulders to the left side. Pull your shoulders back and down, especially your right one. Lift your chin and chest high. Keep your abdominal muscles and buttocks tight and your feet pointed. Stretch your back upward.

Repeat twice with each leg. Now put both feet flat on the floor and stand up slowly. The wind-down is on pages 33–34. Let's go!

SATURDAY #1

Turn to pages 29–33 to warm up with the wind-ups.

Preparatory Position: *Get Ready!*

Lie on your back. Bend your knees toward your chest. Put your knees, ankles, and feet together. Place the palms of your hands on your hamstrings (the back of your thighs). Bend your elbows to the sides. Point your feet. Press the small of your back to the floor. Pull your abdominal muscles down toward your back. Tighten your buttocks and keep them on the floor. Relax your neck, face, and shoulders. Let's go!

1a. Breathe in as you pull your knees down toward your chest with your hands. Rest your head on the floor with your chin inclined toward your chest. Relax your neck, face, and shoulders. Don't lift your buttocks off the floor or separate your knees, ankles, or feet. Press the small of your back to the floor. Pull in your abdominal muscles and tighten your buttocks. Don't drop your elbows to the floor. Keep your feet pointed. Then . . .

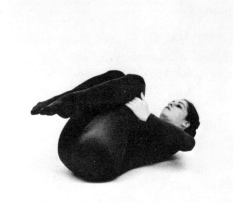

1b. Breathe out as you sit up straight, keeping your knees, ankles, and feet together. Don't let go of your hamstrings. Keep your knees bent toward your chest, your elbows bent to the sides, and your feet pointed. Touch the floor with the tips of your toes. Stretch each vertebra. Hold your chin and chest high. Pull your shoulders back and down. Align your shoulders with your hips. Pull in and tighten. Then point your chin toward your chest. Roll through each vertebra, starting with the base of your spine, to return to the position of 1a. Keep your abdominals and buttocks tight, your feet, knees, and ankles together and your hands on your hamstrings.

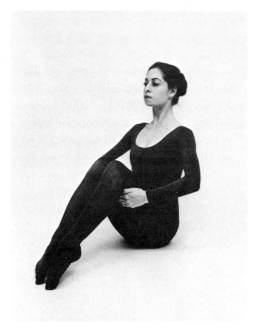

Repeat twice. Finish in the position of 1a for exercise #2.

Preparatory Position: *Get Ready!*

As you lie on your back, raise your arms and legs so that they are perpendicular to the floor. (But if at first you have too much trouble straightening your legs, owing to lack of flexibility and tone, try it with your knees bent.) Turn your legs slightly to the outside. With your heels together, point your feet. Turn the palms of your hands toward your legs. Stretch your fingers and keep them together. Press the small of your back to the floor. Pull your abdominal muscles down toward your back and tighten your buttocks. Relax your neck, face, and shoulders. Let's go!

2a. Breathe in as you flex your feet back at the ankles and split your legs apart. Your legs should still be turned toward the outside. Lower your arms to the floor behind your head with the palms of your hands facing up. Don't separate your fingers. Keep your knees and elbows straight. Relax your neck, face, and shoulders. Tighten your abdominals and buttocks. Stretch your spine long and press the small of your back to the floor.

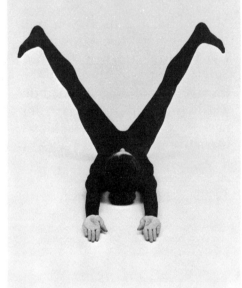

2b. Breathe out as you raise your arms over your torso, crossing them at the wrists. Keep your fingers together. Point your chin toward your chest. Lift your upper back off the floor, aiming your head at your arms. Point your feet. Now, pull your legs together and cross them at the ankles. Don't bend your knees or elbows. Pull in your abdominal muscles and tighten your buttocks. Then return to 2a. Keep your chin inclined toward your chest and your abdominals and buttocks tight. Slowly lower your upper back, neck, and head to the floor.

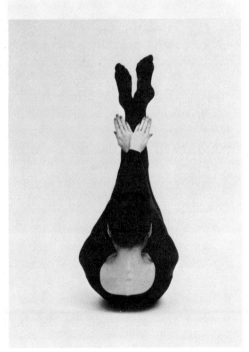

Repeat twice. Then sit up Indian style for the next exercise.

SATURDAY

Preparatory Position: *Get Ready!*

As you sit Indian style, extend your left leg forward in front of your left hip and lift it off the floor. (Your right foot should be crossed above the hamstring of your left leg.) Point your feet. Stretch your arms out to the sides. Turn the palms of your hands down. Stretch your fingers and keep them together. Pull in your abdominal muscles toward your back and up toward your ribs. Pull your weight up off your hips and feel the space between your hips and ribs. Hold your chin and chest high. Pull your shoulders back and down. Don't lean forward or backward. Let's go!

3a. Breathe in as you hold your left leg off the floor in front of your left hip. Flex your left foot back at the ankle. Keep your right foot pointed. Flex your hands back at the wrists. Lift your arms up above your head, pointing your fingers slightly toward the inside. Don't separate your fingers. Keep your elbows straight. Pull in your abdominal muscles and stretch your spine upward. Pull your shoulders back and down. Hold your chin and chest high. Then . . .

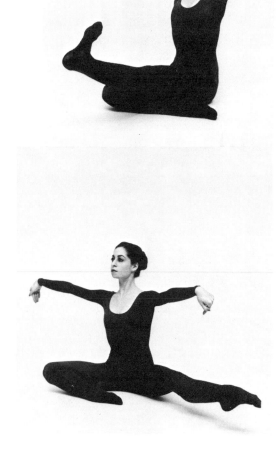

3b. Breathe out as you swing your left leg to the side, pointing your left foot. Your right foot should also still be pointed. Don't move your right leg, bend your left knee, or drop your left leg to the floor. Pull the outer thigh of your right leg toward the floor. Lower your arms to the sides at shoulder level. Don't bend your elbows. Flex your hands forward and point your fingers down. Don't separate your fingers; draw them in toward the palms of your hands. Pull in your abdominal muscles. Don't let your body sag. Pull up out of your torso. Keep your back erect. Don't twist your shoulders; pull them back and down, especially your right one. Hold your chin and chest high. Now return to the position of 3a: Swing your left leg forward and raise your arms above your head.

Repeat twice fluidly and then do this routine with the other leg. Remain seated to do exercise #4.

Preparatory Position: *Get Ready!*

Sit as erect as you can. Stretch your legs straight out in front of you, then slide your right leg to the side. Bend your left knee to the outside, aiming your outer thigh at the floor, and slide your left foot underneath the hamstring of your right leg. Point your feet. Pull your shoulders back and down.

Stretch each vertebra to increase the space between your hips and ribs. Hold your chin and chest high. Pull your abdominal muscles in toward your back and up toward your ribs. Relax your neck. Raise your arms to the sides at shoulder level, with the palms of your hands facing forward. Let's go!

4a. Breathe in as you raise your left arm above your head, turning the palm of your hand toward your right leg. Position your fingers gracefully. Turn your head to the right and look at your right foot. Bend at the waist toward your right leg. Pull both shoulders back and down, especially your left one.

Grab your right ankle with your right hand. Don't move your legs or lift your buttocks off the floor, especially your left side. Hold your chin and chest high. Point your feet. Pull your abdominal muscles in toward your back and up toward your ribs. Tighten your buttocks. Then . . .

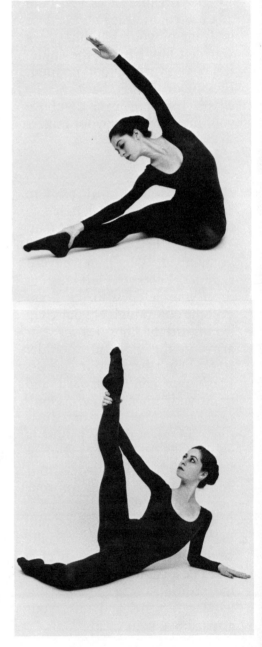

4b. Breathe out as you lower your left arm to your side. Then place your left elbow, forearm, and hand on the floor. (Align your left elbow with your left shoulder.) Lift your right leg up. Don't let go of your right ankle. (But if at first you have difficulty holding onto your ankle as you lift your leg up, hold onto another part of your leg—your calf or knee—or try to stretch your arm as close to your leg as you can.) Raise your leg as high as you can manage. Look at your right leg. Don't change the position of your left leg or bend

your right knee. Point your feet. Don't twist your shoulders. Pull them down and back, especially your left one. Hold your chin and chest high; pull your abdominal muscles in toward your back and tighten your buttocks. Push down onto your left forearm and hand to keep the left side of your torso off the floor. Return to 4a: Push off your left forearm and hand. Stretch your left arm to the side, then lift it above your head. Lower your right leg to the floor with your right hand still gripping your right ankle.

Repeat twice, and then reverse to follow the exercise in the opposite position. Exercise #5 starts in the kneeling position.

SATURDAY

Preparatory Position: *Get Ready!*

From a kneeling position, place your right foot slightly forward and to the right of your right shoulder. Turn your right foot to the outside. Stretch your arms out to the sides at shoulder level, with the palms of your hands facing up. Distribute your weight equally between your right foot and your left knee. (To help you balance, slide your left foot slightly toward the right side.) Point your left foot. Stretch your fingers and keep them together. Tighten your abdominal and buttock muscles. Stretch your spine upward. Pull your shoulders back and down. Hold your chin and chest high. Let's go!

5a. Breathe in as you raise your left arm over your head with the palm of your hand facing right. Don't separate your fingers or bend your elbows. Bend at the waist to the right side. Don't twist your shoulders. Pull them back and down, especially your left one. Touch your right foot with your right hand. Pull in your abdominal muscles and tighten your buttocks. Keep your left foot pointed. Hold your chin and chest high. Then . . .

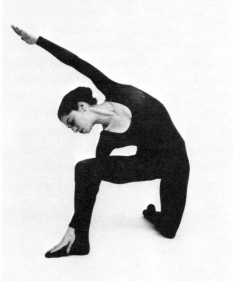

5b. Breathe out as you straighten your back. Pull your weight up, out of your torso. Raise your right arm above your head with the palm of your hand facing to the left. Bend at the waist to the left side. Don't move your legs. Pull your shoulders back and down, especially your right one. Place the palm of your left hand flat on the floor to the left side. Turn your head toward the left and look past your left hand. Pull in and tighten. Keep your left foot pointed. Stretch your fingers and elbows. Hold your chin and chest high.

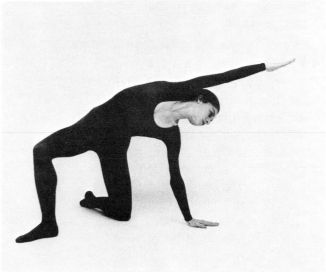

Repeat twice on either knee. For the next exercise, start with both your hands and knees on the floor.

Preparatory Position: *Get Ready!*

Put your knees, ankles, and feet together. Place the palms of your hands directly underneath your shoulders and point your fingers forward. Pull your abdominal muscles in toward your back. Tighten your buttocks. Stretch your spine straight. Push onto the palms of your hands to pull your shoulders down and back. Look straight ahead. Slide your left foot back directly behind your left hip and stretch your left knee. Now lift your left leg off the floor and turn your left leg slightly to the outside. Flex your left foot back at the ankle. Point your right foot. Distribute your weight equally between your hands and your right knee. Let's go!

6a. Breathe in as you lower your left leg. You should feel as if your legs, back, and head are lowering, then lifting (6b), a bucket of nails. Don't bend your left knee. Point both your left and right feet, lightly touching the floor with your left foot. Lower your chin toward your chest. Aim the middle of your back toward the ceiling and your upper and lower back toward the floor. Tighten your abdominal and buttock muscles. Distribute your weight equally between your hands and your right knee, keeping your elbows straight. Then . . .

6b. Breathe out as you lift your left leg up, feeling the resistance. Continue to turn your leg to the outside. Keep your left leg directly behind your left hip. Flex your left foot back at the ankle. Keep your right foot pointed and your left leg and both elbows straight. Lift your chin and chest. Look up. Pull your shoulders back and down. Aim the middle of your back toward the floor and the upper and lower regions of your back toward the ceiling. Pull in your abdominal muscles and tighten your buttocks. Don't lean to either side.

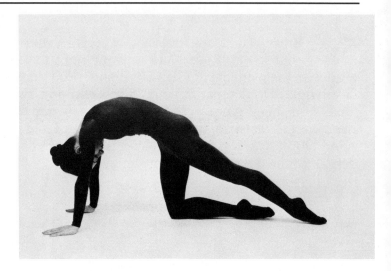

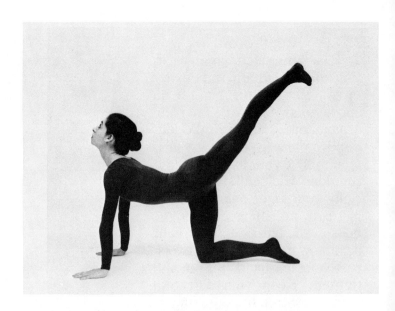

Repeat twice using both legs, then stand up slowly. Now you're ready for exercise #7.

Preparatory Position: *Get Ready!*

Turn your body slightly to the right side and stand erect with your feet together. Be light on your heels. Pull your abdominal muscles in toward your back and up toward your ribs. Stretch your spine upward, pulling your weight off your hips. Hold your chin and chest high. Pull your shoulders back and down. Tighten your buttocks. Stretch your arms out to the sides at shoulder level, with the palms of your hands facing forward. Stretch your fingers and keep them together. Let's go!

7a. Breathe in as you bend your right elbow and swing your right forearm across your chest. Don't drop your right elbow below shoulder level. Keep your left elbow straight and your left arm to the side at shoulder level. Don't separate your fingers. Twist your upper body toward the left side and turn your head also slightly to the left. Lift your left foot and point it next to the calf of your right leg. Bend your right knee. Don't lift your right heel off the floor. Don't tilt your pelvis forward or backward. Keep your back straight! Pull in and tighten. Hold your chin and chest high. Pull your shoulders back and down. Then jump straight off the floor. Turn your body slightly to the left side. Straighten your right elbow, extending your right arm to the side at shoulder level, and swing your left forearm across your chest, being careful to keep your elbow raised. Keep your fingers together. Twist your upper body toward the right side and turn your head slightly to the right. Lift your right foot up, pointing it next to the calf of your left leg. Then . . .

7b. Breathe out as you land softly, rolling toe-to-heel through your left foot. Bend your left knee. Keep your left heel on the floor. Hold your chin and chest high. Don't let your body sag or your fingers separate. Stretch your spine upward. Pull in your abdominal muscles and tighten your buttocks. Pull your shoulders back and down. Now jump off the floor. Turn your body slightly to the right side. Straighten your left elbow, extending your left arm to the side at shoulder level. Land softly in the position of 7a.

Repeat four times at a brisk pace. Stand erect for the next exercise.

Preparatory Position: *Get Ready!*

Standing, place your feet a little wider than shoulder-distance apart, pointing your feet forward. Distribute your weight equally between your feet and incline your weight slightly forward so you are light on your heels. Pull your abdominal muscles in toward your back and up toward your ribs. Tighten your buttocks. Stretch your spine upward and pull your weight up out of your torso. Raise your arms forward with the palms of your hands facing up. Flex your hands back at the wrists. Now bend forward—without bending your knees. Reach through your legs with your hands and put the palms of your hands on the floor. (But if at first it is too difficult for you to stretch forward with or without the palms of your hands on the floor, bend your knees a bit and reach through your legs only as far back and as close to the floor as you can comfortably manage.) Let's go!

8a. Breathe in as you bend your knees, pushing your buttocks to the floor. Don't lift your heels off the floor. Keep your elbows straight and the palms of your hands flat on the floor facing back. Lift your chin and chest upward. Pull your abdominal muscles in toward your back. Pull your shoulders down. Then . . .

8b. Breathe out as you straighten your knees, reaching your buttocks up to the ceiling. Try not to move your hands or feet or bend your elbows. Press your heels on the floor. Lower your head, aiming your chin to your chest. Look through your legs. Pull in your abdominals and tighten your buttocks. Relax your neck, face, and shoulders.

Repeat twice fluidly. Finish in the position of 8b. Then bend your knees and roll up through each vertebra to stand erect. You're ready for exercise #9.

SATURDAY

Preparatory Position: *Get Ready!*

Standing with your feet placed a little wider than shoulder-distance apart and pointing forward, bend forward from your hips without bending your knees. Don't arch or curve your spine. Place the palms of your hands on the floor. Walk forward on your hands until your heels are just about to lift off the floor. Keep your knees and elbows straight. Reach your buttocks to the ceiling. Lower your head, aiming your chin to your chest. Look through your legs. Pull your abdominal muscles in toward your back. Tighten your buttocks. Stretch your spine. Relax your neck, face, and shoulders. (But if you have trouble doing this exercise at this time because you can't straighten your knees, do it with your knees bent.) Let's go!

9a. Breathe in as you walk forward on your hands, keeping your knees and back straight. Don't move your feet. Push your hips toward the floor. Lift your chin up. Push down onto your hands to pull your shoulders down and back. Pull in your abdominal muscles and tighten your buttocks. Stretch your elbows. Then . . .

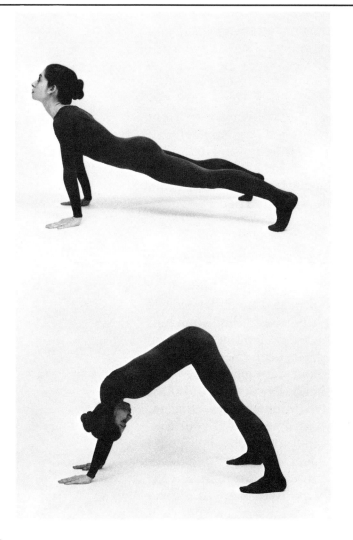

9b. Breathe out as you walk backward on your hands, just until your heels are down on the floor. Keep your knees and back straight. Push your buttocks toward the ceiling. Lower your head, aiming your chin to your chest. Look through your legs. Stretch your spine long. Don't bend your elbows. Pull in your abdominal muscles and tighten your buttocks.

Repeat twice. Then put your feet together. Walk backward on your hands, bringing them close to your feet. Bend your knees and stand up slowly. Turn the page to do the last exercise of today's session.

*If you've never exercised before or are very much out of shape, omit this exercise the first week.

SATURDAY

Preparatory Position: *Get Ready!*

Put your legs together and stand straight. Bend your knees, keeping them together, and place your fingertips in front of you on the floor. From this squatting position, slide your left foot back directly behind your left hip. Straighten your left knee. Point your left foot and press your right heel on the floor. Then lower your left knee to the floor. Pull your abdominal muscles in toward your back and up toward your ribs. Tighten your buttocks. Pull your shoulders back and down. Chin and chest high! Let's go!

10a. Breathe in as you shift your weight forward onto your fingertips. Don't move your hands or your left knee. Keep your right heel on the floor and your left foot pointed. Push your hips forward. Lean over your right thigh. Stretch your spine. Don't bend your elbows. Hold your chin and chest high. Pull your shoulders back and down. Pull in and tighten. Then . . .

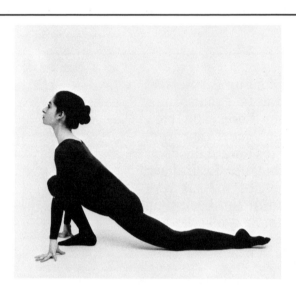

10b. Breathe out as you shift your weight backward onto the palms of your hands, placed at either side of your right foot. Pull your hips backward, then sit down on your left heel. Bend forward over your right leg, aiming your forehead toward your shin. Stretch your elbows, fingers, and right knee. Point your feet. Relax your neck, face, and shoulders. Pull in your abdominal muscles and tighten your buttocks. Return to 10a: Bend your right knee. Place your right foot flat on the floor. Shift your weight forward.

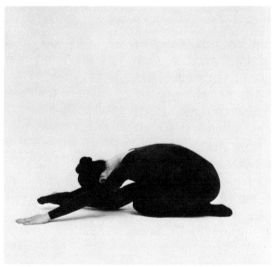

Repeat twice, alternating legs. Then put both feet on the floor, bend your knees, and stand up slowly. Now turn to pages 33–34 to do the wind-down.

SUNDAY

Let's get set for today's session: Turn to pages 29–33 and do the wind-up exercises. Then sit down.

Preparatory Position: *Get Ready!*

Sit with your legs spread apart. Extend your arms at shoulder level in front of you. Turn the palms of your hands up. Flex your feet back at the ankles.

Hold your chin and chest high. Pull your abdominal muscles in toward your back and up toward your ribs. Tighten your buttocks. Stretch your spine upward and pull your weight up out of your torso. Pull your shoulders back and down. Let's go!

1a. Breathe in as you point your feet and aim your small toes at the floor. Straighten your knees. With the palms of your hands facing up, close your fingers into tight fists. Bend your elbows inward and bring your fists to either side of your chest. Pull your shoulders back and down. Lean back. Press your legs to the floor. Lower your head toward your chest. Pull in your abdominal muscles and tighten your buttocks. Then . . .

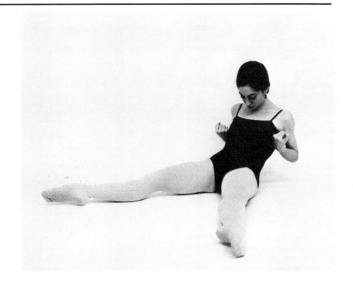

1b. Breathe out as you flex your feet back at the ankles. Don't move your legs! Now, bend your knees, pushing your kneecaps toward the ceiling. Straighten your elbows and raise your arms above your head. Spread your fingers apart and turn the palms of your hands forward. Lean forward, stretching your spine. Lift your chin and chest. Pull in your abdominal muscles and tighten your buttocks.

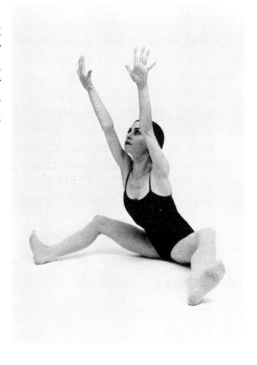

Repeat twice. Stay seated for exercise #2.

SUNDAY

Preparatory Position: *Get Ready!*

Start in a sitting position with your legs together. Bend your knees, sliding your feet flat on the floor toward your buttocks. Keep your knees, feet, and ankles together. Place your hands on the floor behind your torso, slightly wider than shoulder-distance apart. Turn each hand to the outside. Pull your abdominal muscles in toward your back and up toward your ribs. Tighten your buttocks. Hold your chin and chest high. Pull your shoulders back and down. Let's go!

2a. Breathe in as you lower your forehead to your knees. Don't move your hands. Flex your feet back at the ankles. Don't separate your knees, ankles, or feet. Pull your shoulders down. Pull in your abdominal muscles and tighten your buttocks. Relax your neck, shoulders, and face. Then . . .

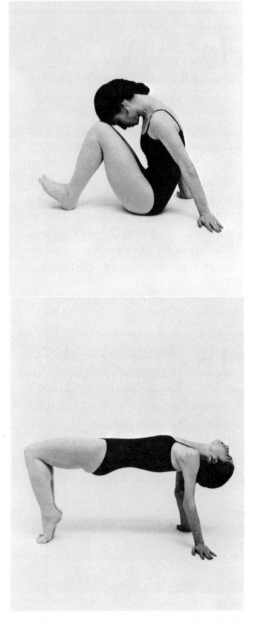

2b. Breathe out as you push down onto the palms of your hands and straighten your elbows. Lift your buttocks off the floor. Raise your hips, thighs, and chest toward the ceiling. Keep your knees, ankles, and feet together. Rise onto the balls of your feet. Pull your shoulders back and down. Lift your chin and lower your head back. Pull in your abdominal muscles. Tighten your buttocks. Then lower your buttocks and heels to the floor. Bring your head forward.

Repeat twice. Remain seated for the next exercise.

SUNDAY

Preparatory Position: *Get Ready!*

From a sitting position, start with your legs straight out in front of you. Press them together and point your feet. Pull your abdominal muscles in toward your back and up toward your ribs. Pull your shoulders back and down. Tighten your buttocks. Pull your weight up out of your torso. Hold your chin and chest high. Now place your fingers on top of your shoulders. Let's go!

3a. Breathe in as you sit erect, stretching each vertebra. (Your shoulders should be directly above your hips.) Don't move your hands. Lift your elbows above shoulder level, aiming them out to the sides. Straighten your knees. Keep your feet pointed, your legs together, your chin and chest high, your abdominals and buttocks tight, and your shoulders back and down. Then . . .

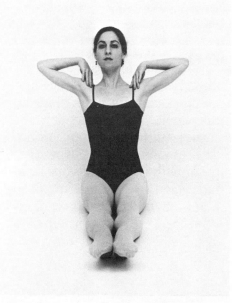

3b. Breathe out as you bend your right knee and press your right outer thigh to the floor. Point your right foot next to the calf of your left leg. Twist your left shoulder forward and your right shoulder back. Bend forward from your waist. Keep your fingers on your shoulders and your chin and chest high. Touch your left elbow to your right foot while lifting your right elbow toward the ceiling. Look at your right foot. Don't move your left leg! Keep your left knee straight and your left foot pointed. Pull in and tighten.

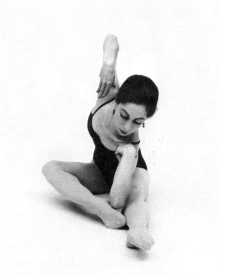

Repeat four times at a quick pace, alternating legs and shoulders. Finish in the position of 3a for exercise #4.

SUNDAY

Preparatory Position: *Get Ready!*

As you sit with your legs straight out in front of you, extend your right arm forward and your left arm out to the side at shoulder level, with the palms of your hands facing down. Position your fingers gracefully. Stretch each vertebra, starting at the base of your spine. Lift your weight up and out of your torso. Pull your abdominal muscles in toward your back and up toward your ribs. Pull your shoulders back and down. Hold your chin and chest high. Point your feet. Tighten your buttocks. Feel as if you are doing this exercise underwater; create resistance for your arms and legs to move against. Let's go!

4a. Breathe in as you flex your feet back at the ankles. Bend your right knee and touch your right outer thigh to the floor. Keep your left leg straight in front of your left hip and shoulder. Touch your left thigh with the heel of your right foot. Don't let your arms drop below shoulder level or your elbows bend. Bring your left arm forward and your right arm out to the side. Pull in your abdominal muscles and tighten your buttocks. Hold your chin and chest high. Pull your shoulders back and down, especially your right one. Keep your back straight; your shoulders should be directly above your hips. Then . . .

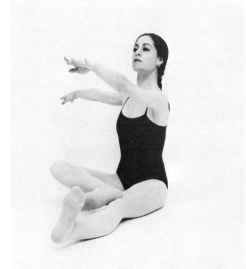

4b. Breathe out as you point your feet. Straighten your right leg out to the side and hold it off the floor. Don't bend your left knee or move your left leg. At shoulder level, bring your right arm forward and your left arm to the side. Don't change the position of your fingers. Stretch your elbows. Pull in your abdominal muscles and tighten your buttocks. Your back should be perpendicular to the floor. Lift your ribs up, away from your hips. Hold your chest and chin high. Pull your shoulders back and down, especially your left one.

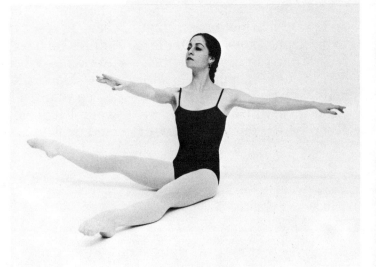

Repeat twice, alternating sides. Then stand up slowly for exercise #5.

*If you've never exercised before or are very much out of shape, omit this exercise the first week.

100

SUNDAY

Preparatory Position: *Get Ready!*

Stand with your right foot about 12″ in front of your left. Turn your legs slightly to the outside. Distribute your weight equally on both feet. Stretch your arms behind you. Interlace your fingers, with the palms of your hands facing your back. Pull your abdominal muscles in toward your back and up toward your ribs. Tighten your buttocks. Pull your shoulders back and down. Now bend forward. Lower your forehead toward your right leg. (If straightening your elbows with your fingers interlaced, or straightening your knees, is too difficult for you at this time, don't strain yourself. Work up to the more difficult exercises slowly.) Let's go!

5a. Breathe in as you bend your knees. Don't move your feet, lift your heels off the floor, or separate your hands. Bend your elbows, lifting them upward. Bring your hands to the middle of your back. Pull in and tighten. Pull your shoulders back and down. Relax your back, ankles, neck, face, and toes. Continue to point your forehead at your right leg. Then . . .

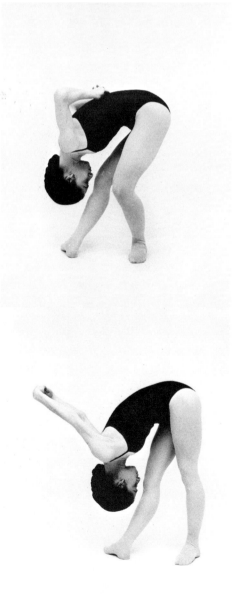

5b. Breathe out as you straighten your knees and stretch your elbows. Move your arms down toward your head. Keep your legs turned to the outside and your fingers together! Pull your abdominal muscles in and tighten your buttocks. Don't twist your shoulders. Pull them back. Relax your back, neck, face, and toes. Try to touch your right leg with your forehead.

Repeat twice fluidly to each side. Then slowly stand erect to do exercise #6.

SUNDAY

Preparatory Position: *Get Ready!*

Stand straight with your legs together. Distribute your weight equally on both feet. Be light on your heels! Pull in your abdominal muscles. Tighten your buttocks. Pull your shoulders back and down. Hold your chest and chin high. Stretch each vertebra upward. Extend your arms forward at shoulder level. Interlace your fingers. Turn the palms of your hands away from you. Let's go!

6a. Breathe in as you bend your knees. Keep your toes, heels, and knees together and your heels on the floor. Lower your arms. Don't bend your elbows or separate your fingers. Then . . .

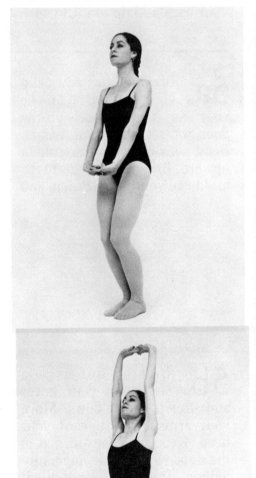

6b. Jump off the floor. Point your feet. Stretch your knees. Raise your arms above your head. Keep your elbows straight and your fingers interlaced. Turn your legs slightly to the outside. Your legs should be about 12″ apart. Keep your back straight. Pull in your abdominal muscles and tighten your buttocks. Hold your chin and chest high. Pull your shoulders back and down. Then . . .

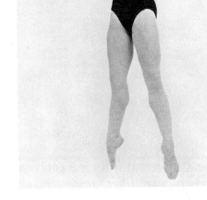

6c. Breathe out as you land. With your legs still turned to the outside, you should roll from the balls of your feet through your heels to cushion your landing. Put your heels together, aiming your toes toward the sides. Bend your knees. Don't lift your heels off the floor or separate your fingers. Keep your back straight and your arms above your head. (Your shoulders and arms should be aligned with your hips.) Pull in your abdominal muscles and tighten your buttocks. Hold your chin and chest high. Pull your shoulders back and down. Then jump off the floor (6b). Turn your legs to the inside, bringing your toes, heels, and knees together. Lower your arms and land in the position of 6a.

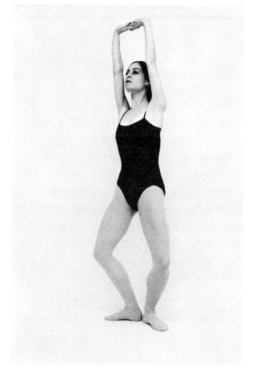

Repeat four times at a brisk pace. Finish in the position of 6a for the next exercise.

SUNDAY

Preparatory Position: *Get Ready!*

As you stand with your legs, heels, and toes together, raise your arms above your head. Stretch your fingers but keep them together. Flex your hands back at the wrists. Turn the palms of your hands up and point your fingers toward each other. Bend your elbows, aiming them out to the sides. Bend your knees and press them together. Keep your heels on the floor. Pull your abdominal muscles in toward your back and up toward your ribs. Tighten your buttocks. Pull your shoulders back and down. Hold your chin and chest high. Stretch each vertebra upward. Pull your weight up off your hips. Let's go!

7a. Breathe in as you bend at the waist to the right side. Don't bend forward or backward. Turn your head to the right. Keep your knees bent, your knees, ankles, and feet together, and your heels on the floor. Don't separate your fingers. Lift your weight up out of your torso. Pull in your abdominal muscles. Tighten your buttocks. Hold your chin and chest high. Don't twist your shoulders. Pull them back and down, especially your left one. Then . . .

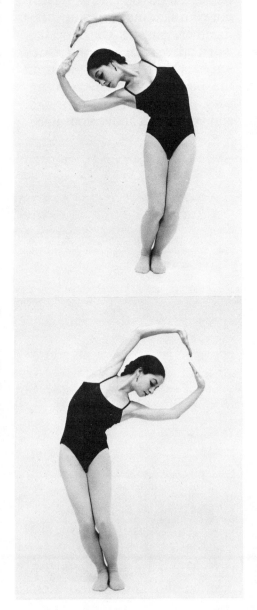

7b. Breathe out as you bend at the waist to the left side. Keep your knees bent. Don't separate your knees, ankles, or feet. Don't lift your heels off the floor. Aim your elbows out to the sides. Stretch your fingers. Turn your head to the left. Pull in and tighten. Don't let your body sag. Hold your chin and chest high. Pull your shoulders back and down, especially your right one.

Repeat twice at a quick pace, alternating sides. Then lie down on your left side to do exercise #8.

Preparatory Position: *Get Ready!*

Lying on your left side, stretch your left arm along the floor, the palm of your left hand facing up. Rest your head on top of your left arm. Stretch your right arm past your right ear so that you can place the palms of your hands together. Bend your left knee along the floor and move it slightly forward to help you balance. Straighten your right leg to align it with your hips, shoulders, and arms. Point your feet. Bend your elbows, aiming them toward the sides. Place your right hand on top of your left elbow and your left hand on top of your right elbow. Relax your neck and face. Pull your shoulders back. Keep your back straight. (It's helpful to tilt your hips slightly forward.) Pull your abdominal muscles in toward your back. Tighten your buttocks. (You should be in the position of 8b.) Let's go!

8a. Breathe in as you flex your right foot back at the ankle. Rotate your right leg slightly to the outside; aim your toes up to the ceiling. Lift your right leg. Keep your right knee straight and your right leg in the same plane with your hips, shoulders, and elbows. Point your left foot. Don't move your left leg or your arms. Pull in your abdominal muscles and tighten your buttocks. Keep your spine straight and your shoulders back. Relax your neck and face. Then . . .

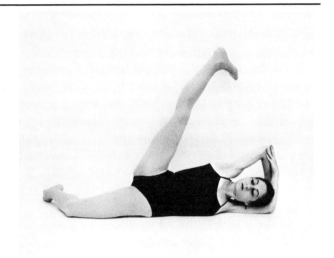

8b. Breathe out as you point your right foot. Rotate your right leg to the inside; aim the inside of your foot to the floor. Keep your left foot pointed. Lower your right leg. Don't move your left leg or bend your right knee. Don't change the alignment of your body; your hips, shoulders, elbows, and right leg should form a straight line. Pull in and tighten. Don't twist your shoulders. Don't move your arms. Relax your neck and face.

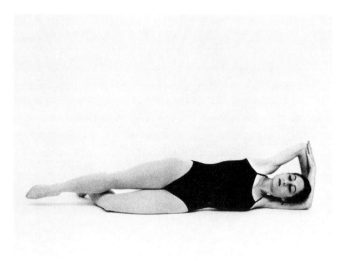

Repeat twice on both sides. Then roll onto your back for the next exercise.

Preparatory Position: *Get Ready!*

Lying on your back, bend your knees toward your chest and then straighten them so that your legs are perpendicular to the floor. Cross your left ankle over your right. Turn your legs slightly to the outside. Point your feet. Pull your abdominal muscles in toward your back. Tighten your buttocks. Interlace your fingers behind your head. Rest your elbows, neck, head, and shoulders on the floor. Point your chin toward your chest. Relax your face. Let's go!

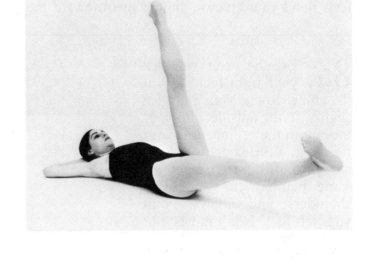

9a. Breathe in as you flex your feet back at the ankles. Hold your left leg up. Lower your right leg toward the floor. Your legs should still be turned to the outside. Don't bend your knees. (But if you can't straighten your knees at this time, do the exercise with your knees bent.) Point your chin toward your chest. Rest your head, elbows, neck, and shoulders on the floor. Keep your fingers interlaced. Pull in your abdominal muscles and tighten your buttocks. Press the small of your back to the floor. Then . . .

9b. Breathe out as you point your feet. Don't move your left leg. Lift your right leg up next to your left leg. Cross your legs at the ankles. Stretch your knees. Turn your legs toward the outside. Pull your elbows together. With the help of your hands, lift your head, neck, and upper back off the floor toward your legs. Don't change the position of your hands. Press your chin on your chest. Relax your face. Tighten your abdominals and buttocks. Return to 9a: open your elbows and lower your upper back, neck, head, elbows, and right leg toward the floor.

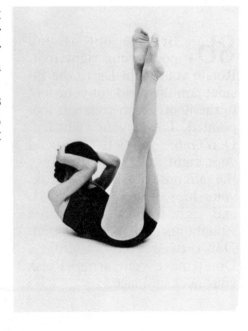

Repeat twice in both leg positions. Now lie down on your stomach to do the last exercise of today's session.

Preparatory Position: *Get Ready!*

Lying on your stomach, stretch your legs and arms along the floor, making a straight line with your body. Then place your right hand on top of your left and cross your right ankle on top of your left ankle. Point your feet. Stretch your knees. Bend your elbows and slide your hands in toward your head. Rest your forehead on top of your hands. Relax your neck, face, shoulders, and fingers. Pull your abdominal muscles up toward your back. Tighten your buttocks. Let's go!

10a. Breathe in as you lift your right leg off the floor directly behind your right shoulder and hip. Keep your forehead on your hands and your elbows, left leg, hands, and chest resting on the floor. Point your feet. Stretch your knees. Don't twist your hips. Press them on the floor. Relax your fingers, neck, face, and shoulders. Pull in your abdominal muscles and tighten your buttocks.

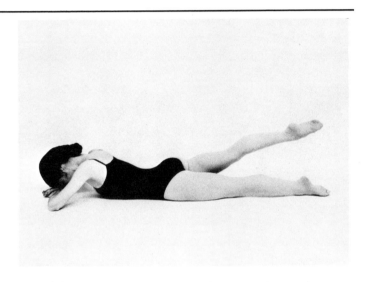

10b. Breathe out as you push down onto your hands, stretching your elbows. Lift your chin and chest away from the floor. Look up to the ceiling. Pull your shoulders back and down. Don't bend your knees or move your hands. Cross your legs at the ankles just off the floor: lift your left leg up to your right leg and lower your right leg down to your left leg. Pull in your abdominal muscles. Tighten your buttocks. Keep your feet pointed and your hips on the floor.

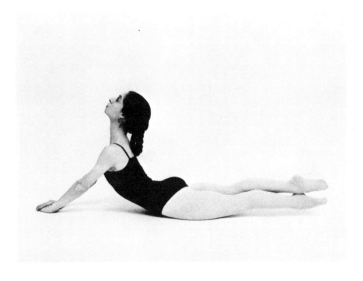

Repeat twice, alternating legs. Then stand up slowly. Let's cool down. Turn to pages 33-34 and do the wind-down exercise.

Chapter 8

THE ST. TROPEZ
BODY PLAN

The St. Tropez Body Plan is an extra provision of the French Riviera Body Program. It's a more advanced version: you do two consecutive days' sessions, plus the wind-up and wind-down exercises with each session. Of course, the French Riviera Body Program's Basic Rules and Special Tips are applicable and the benefits are the same, if not greater.

On the St. Tropez Body Plan, you merge . . .

Monday with Tuesday
Tuesday with Wednesday
Wednesday with Thursday
Thursday with Friday
Friday with Saturday
Saturday with Sunday
Sunday with Monday

As always, start with the wind-ups, then do that day's session and the wind-down. Then, do the wind-ups again, followed by the *next* day's session and the wind-down. For example, if it's Monday, do the wind-ups, Monday's session, and the wind-down. Then do the wind-ups once again, but go on to Tuesday's session afterward and finish with the wind-down. Because it takes fives minutes to complete each day's session, including, of course, the wind-up and wind-down exercises, your exercise periods on the St. Tropez Body Plan will be at least ten minutes long. (Keep this in mind when you're scheduling your exercise periods.)

On the St. Tropez Body Plan, you do more exercises and you exercise for greater lengths of time. So don't start it until you've been on the French Riviera Body Program for *at least* four weeks. It's safer for you and better for your body if

you wait until you're ready to intensify and lengthen your exercise periods under this accelerated program. It will be easier for you to learn the sessions, too.

You should go on the St. Tropez Body Plan only if . . .

• You've been on the French Riviera Body Program for at least four weeks.
• You can do all the exercises without modification.
• You are so familiar with each exercise, you no longer find it necessary to stop and read the instructions.
• You know the sequence of each session so well you can go from one exercise to the next without hesitation.
• You can complete each of the seven sessions from wind-up to wind-down in five minutes.
• You are capable of doing each of the seven sessions from wind-up to wind-down twice through during an exercise period within ten minutes.

Now once you're following the St. Tropez Body Plan, be sure to approach the sessions—especially the second day's—with the same care you used when you were following a single day's exercise session each day.

Why the St. Tropez Body Plan? Why didn't I call this provision the St. Raphaël Body Plan or the Cannes Body Plan? In many ways, St. Tropez is a typical Provençal village, with its red roof tops, its old streets and squares, and its sun-drenched Mediterranean climate. But ever since Brigitte Bardot made it her home, St. Tropez has become one of France's most popular resorts, a favorite spot of the jet set and a world-famous luxury port.

St. Tropez has a particular fascination. It's no wonder why. Especially from June to September, St. Tropez explodes with stunning people who have the French Riviera Body, people who enjoy life and utilize their high energy, great condition, and self-confidence to the fullest. There's lots to see. Topless sunbathing, which is said to have originated at Tahiti Plage in St. Tropez, is prevalent. And there's lots to do. Whether waterskiing, dancing, boating, or playing tennis, French Riviera Body People are where it all happens. Day or night, the fun never stops.

St. Tropez is an extraordinarily exciting place. There, the reasons to exercise regularly and the benefits of exercising daily are accentuated even more than at most of the other glamorous locations along the French Riviera. And that's why naming this amplified edition of the French Riviera Body Program the St. Tropez Body Plan seemed so right.

Chapter 9

MORE ANSWERS
TO QUESTIONS

Here are more answers to questions about the French Riviera Body Program—answers to questions such as these: "Why can't we add, subtract, or substitute exercises?"; "If I don't have much time, can I do half a session and do the other half later?"; "What if I do this program every other day? Will the program still work?"; "Is there a point at which you reach a plateau?"; "Will the program still work if I don't exercise during the weekends?"; "I just started the program and it's taking me a lot longer than five minutes to do the days' sessions from the wind-ups to the wind-down. What am I doing wrong?"; "You talk so much about flexibility, coordination, strength, and stamina. What do they have to do with looking good?"; "How long will it take me to get back into shape?"; and "What do you mean by 'optimum,' 'excellent,' and 'very good' results?"

This chapter will be helpful to you before you start this program. You'll also find it particularly useful after you're underway.

Q. *Why are there seven 5-minute exercise sessions instead of, for example, one workout to follow for forty-five to sixty minutes?*
A. I don't think long workouts in exercise books are very realistic. It's difficult to exercise for long periods of time on your own and do the same exercises every day without getting bored. And boredom is an enemy. It can destroy marriages, vacations, and exercise programs. So who needs it?

Instead of making a book with just one workout to follow for a traditional all-or-nothing, heavy-duty, sweat-it-out exercise period, I formulated the French Riviera Body Program so you could truly want to and be able to follow a daily exercise program for a lifetime, in Monte Carlo or in your bedroom.

The chances of completing each 5-minute session are great. The requirement of exercising daily is a practical one, to promote consistency, but it's easy to exercise several times a day and the motivation to exercise for longer periods of time is encouraged. And, in order to complete each session within five minutes, you're compelled to exercise at a nonstop, vigorous pace, which contributes to cardiovascular fitness.

When goals are modest—for example, striving to complete a day's session from wind-up to wind-down in five minutes—the probability of not only reaching your goal but surpassing it is high. Being in control of your own exercise methods is part of this program's image-building process. Discovering from experience that you can exercise and get fabulous results (as you can on this program) is motivational and encouraging.

Q. *Why do you suggest we follow this program more than once a day?*
A. By spreading out your exercise time during the day—as opposed to doing one long exercise period—it's easier to approach the program with a fresh outlook and to be concerned with the quality of the exercise session. For many people, it's the most convenient way to exercise and, in some cases, the only way in which they can adhere to a regular exercise program. They may not have all the time they'd like to spend following a program such as this at any one given time per day. And doing my fitness-packed exercises several times a day keeps your body active, often stimulating it to release beta morphines which give you a sense of euphoria.

Q. *Why do you say we should exercise every day when some say, to give an example, that thirty minutes of exercise three or four times a week is satisfactory?*
A. The French Riviera Body Program reflects my years of experience as a dancer, ballet and exercise teacher, and author as well as all the research, interviewing, and traveling I did for this book. It also takes into account the most recent findings of doctors and scientists: Daily exercise is a necessity for the body. It's the easiest and surest way to get in shape and make exercise a habit. And the length and intensity of one's exercise period is not nearly as important as how regularly it is done.

When you exercise every day, you get fast and lasting results. You don't lose ground as you may by exercising only every couple of days. For example, when you exercise daily, stiffness doesn't disrupt your flexibility. On the French Riviera Body Program, you progress continually; each day you build on the previous day's accomplishments, and exercising becomes a natural part of your everyday life. It's a guaranteed way to get in shape, and to stay in shape, too.

Q. *Why can't we add, subtract, or substitute exercises? Why can't we do an exercise from one day's session in addition to or as a substitute for an exercise from another day's session?*
A. When you start playing around with the exercises and sessions—adding, subtracting, substituting—you quickly lose the momentum, ease, structure, and control that are the hallmarks of this program. For example, to add Monday's session on to Saturday's, subtract half of Sunday's session and postpone it till Tuesday, take exercise #3 from Wednesday and repeat it after Friday's session . . . is to follow an unbalanced program of your own, one in which getting any results is a gamble. More importantly, once you permit yourself to stray from the program as it has been expressly designed, you are more likely to take other shortcuts, as convenience dictates, until you're no longer on this program at all.

I designed each session like a recipe, with the proper ingredients to produce the French Riviera Body. In any other form, the sessions would not be as effective. The French Riviera Body Program was designed to help you look great and feel terrific. So why would you want to change anything?

Q. *Why must the exercises be practiced in the exact order given in each session?*

A. The sessions were constructed so you could exercise thoroughly, enjoy a variety of movements, and get great results fast. The order in which the exercises were arranged—almost "choreographed" like a dance—enables you to follow them easily and smoothly so you can accomplish the most in the least amount of time and with the minimum expenditure of energy.

For maximum results, it's necessary both physiologically and psychologically to do the exercises in their established order.

Q. *Sometimes my toes cramp while I'm exercising. What should I do?*
A. Shake your feet, rub and massage your toes and the balls of your feet, and keep going. During the day—whenever you have the chance—exercise your feet, ankles, and toes as described in the wind-up chapter on page 29. These exercises will improve the circulation of the blood flowing through your feet and toes and increase their flexibility and strength.

This problem is not uncommon and it occurs as a result of stimulating and toning the feet and toes in many ways those areas aren't used to. Once your feet and toes become accustomed to being exercised, these bouts of foot cramps will diminish.

Also, check the fit of your shoes and hosiery: Are they too tight? Do they constrict the circulation of your blood in your feet and toes? Correct these situations immediately. Wear more comfortable shoes and hosiery.

Q. *Will the facial exercises given in the wind-up chapter tighten my skin?*
A. Facial exercises do not create the kind of dramatic changes—the reproportioning and increased strength and flexibility—that the other exercises in this program produce, but you can expect your skin to look and stay healthier, more radiant, more youthful and resilient.

Q. *If people are already engaged in other exercise, sport, or dance programs why do they need this one?*
A. The program they may be engaged in may not be as substantive as the French Riviera Body Program, which contains movements to increase strength, stamina, and flexibility, and to improve shape, coordination, balance, and more. "I need something more than ballet. It doesn't do everything for my body," said one of my exercise students who is a ballet dancer. "I find that your exercises work muscles which aren't worked

enough in ballet, like the abdominals and the backs of the legs. Since I've started doing your exercises, I've gone down a couple of inches, my extension is higher, and I'm much stronger." Many activities are inconvenient to do daily or must be performed at a specific location to make use of equipment, for instance. And for too many people, the program they're following may be incompatible with their financial status, making getting in shape a double strain on them.

For others the French Riviera Body 5-Minute, 7-Day Exercise Sessions could work well as warm-ups. Most injuries are caused by tired, cold, or inflexible muscles and joints. By following this program, one can thoroughly prepare one's body for the movements involved in other activities. "I run. Before and after running, I do your exercises," said another student of mine. "Before running I use your exercises as a warm-up and afterwards I like to stretch out with them."

Q. *Sometimes when I skip a few days, my muscles begin to twitch and I feel sluggish and tense. Why?*
A. Congratulations! You need to exercise. Your body has developed a very healthy addiction to feeling and looking good, burning off excess adrenaline and anxiety, and having energy when you exercise regularly.

Your body expects to be exercised with certain exercises on certain days. When you don't follow this program as you should, your body, like a good friend, is going to remind you that you must.

Q. *I can't do any of the exercises the way you can: I can't straighten my knees, bend as far to the side, lift my leg up as high. Do you think I'll ever be able to do them as you do?*
A. Without any doubt you will become more flexible, which means you *could* ultimately be more flexible than I am. But how far, high, how straight, how much your body can bend, reach, jump, or kick—now or ever—does not affect how you benefit from the exercises.

It's doing the best you can and following this program exactly as it is written that determines whether or not you become more flexible, not your present abilities or how terrific you look exercising.

Don't forget: I started bending, stretching, straightening my knees, and so on as a toddler. It should be no wonder that I can lift my leg high or touch my toes. And now I'm your personal exercise teacher. It's my joy and responsibility to give you the clearest and most correct example of my fitness-packed exercises so you have a good example to follow and something to aim for.

Enjoy your period of exercise. Look at me as you would look at a model in a magazine: someone to show you how to do something to look your best. Your best, not hers or his.

We all have our own peak. Go for yours!

Q. *I just started the program and it's taking me a lot longer than five minutes to do each day's session from wind-up to wind-down. What am I doing wrong?*
A. Nothing. Of course it's taking you longer. You've never done these exercises before. And you've got instructions and rules to read and pictures to study. But within a short time—approximately two weeks—you should be able to complete each day's session within five minutes. However, you shouldn't feel compelled to; you can take as long as you need or want.

Q. *Because I don't know this program well enough, I can't seem to follow the sessions without having to stop between exercises. Am I still getting the benefits of this program?*
A. Not knowing the exercises and having to do them in a stop-and-go manner are parts of the process of beginning the French Riviera Body Program. This stopping and going to learn the exercises obliges you to start this program gradually so you will accumulate the benefits rather than discouraging thoughts and sore muscles.

Q. *Will I get to know the sessions well enough to do them without reading the instructions?*
A. Within a few weeks you'll only have to refer to the text once in a while. You will be very familiar with the exercises and the sequence of each session. But once you reach this point, look over the text every two weeks to make sure you're following this program exactly as described.

Before you start this program, it is advisable to study the exercises by reading the text and examining the accompanying pictures to familiarize yourself with the movements and the order in which they are laid out. That will help you learn the program faster.

Q. *If I don't have much time, can I do half a session now and do the other half later?*
A. If you are really pressed for time, do only one repetition of each exercise but do all the exercises—the wind-up, the wind-down, and the day's

or days' sessions—to receive the full benefits from your exercise periods. You need to and you must. That's the only way this program works.

The sessions are well-balanced body treatments but only when you do all the exercises. It's the contents of each exercise and the combination of exercises making up the days' sessions that lead to the development and maintenance of the French Riviera Body—but only when they are followed on their appropriate days and in their assigned sequences!

To do one half a session or anything other than what has been specified is to waste your time and energy and deny yourself the French Riviera Body.

Q. *Must I do the wind-up if I only have a few minutes to exercise?*
A. Yes. The body moves more smoothly and is more receptive to the benefits of the days' sessions after it goes through the wind-ups.

Q. *Should I time how long it takes me to do the wind-up, the day's session, and the wind-down?*
A. Timing your exercise periods, especially upon beginning this program, is a good idea. At first, doing all the exercises from the wind-up chapter, the day's session, and the wind-down will probably take you longer than five minutes to complete. So knowing how much time you need to exercise will enable you to make a practical schedule of your exercise periods. Keeping track of how much time you are spending to exercise will also help you know how to vary the pace of the exercises and govern how much time you can spend on each exercise and still complete all of them within the desired five-minute period. Ultimately, the speed and ease with which you do the exercises will tell you if you are ready to go on to the St. Tropez Body Plan.

Q. *What do you mean by optimum, excellent, very good, and good results?*
A. Since it's natural to wonder how fast this program works, I labeled the results optimum, excellent, very good, and good to indicate how soon, approximately, it will be possible to enjoy the benefits of this program.

If you follow this program exactly as described for 30–40 minutes every day you can get optimum results. That means you could start to see and feel yourself getting the French Riviera Body in as little as two weeks. If you follow this program for 20–30 minutes, 10–20 minutes, or 5–10 minutes a day, it could take anywhere from two and a half weeks to two months before you start to see and feel yourself achieving the French Riviera Body.

Q. *Can I exercise, for example, five minutes in the morning, ten minutes in the afternoon, and fifteen minutes at night? In other words, can I exercise for different lengths of time throughout the day and different amounts of time each day?*
A. Yes to both questions as long as you exercise every day and recognize how much exercising is required to accomplish your goals.

On the French Riviera Body Program, as you know, how long you exercise, when, where, and with whom you do it are decided by you. It's best, though, for both your physical and mental well-being, not to cram in a lot of exercising one day and very little the next. Ideally, you should try to regulate your exercise schedule so you exercise a certain amount of time each day and, if possible, at the same times each day, to make exercise part of your daily and weekly routines. To help you, I have included a chart for you to fill in with your own schedule. Use it!

Q. *I can follow this program quite easily Monday through Friday, but when it comes to the weekends, I really can't seem to get myself to exercise or make a schedule for it. My weekends are so unpredictable—I don't know what I'm doing until I do it. Will the program still work if I don't follow it on the weekends?*
A. This program works best when you follow it as specified. And that means exercising daily even over the weekends or whenever you have a day off or holiday.

One of the reasons you may have trouble getting yourself to exercise over the weekends or even making a schedule for it is that you probably practice the philosophy that days off—holidays, weekends—should be more spontaneous, fun, and relaxing than the weekdays. But to think or live that way should make no difference in how you behave toward your body and the French Riviera Body Program. After all, during the weekends, your body doesn't stop wanting and needing to be kept healthy and fit, so why should you deny it its rightful condition?

This program has to be part of every day and it can be. Remember, it adjusts to your lifestyle, needs, schedules, and goals. During the weekend, you don't have to exercise for the same lengths of time, at the same hours or locations, or for the same specific reasons as during the week.

Treat each day individually, particularly your days off. If you find it impossible or undesirable to keep up with the same sort of exercise schedule as you keep during the week, or you can't seem to schedule one for the weekends—don't. You'll only discourage yourself from exercising at all.

Don't put so much pressure on yourself. Relax and enjoy your weekends by doing this program at a comfortable pace, time, and location that suits your weekend or holiday plans—or lack of them—and your moods. Let this program work for you and with you. Follow this program when it's convenient so you can and will exercise!

Never think that if you exercise less than you do during the week, it's not worth doing at all. It's not how long you exercise but that you do it every day, accumulating your achievements, that brings you closer to attaining, then keeping the French Riviera Body.

Q. *But I really don't have time to exercise every day. What if I do it every other day? Will the program still work?*
A. As you know, this program was designed to help you achieve the French Riviera Body. And it works—you can and will attain it, but only by following this program exactly as described, without variations.

The excuse that you don't have the time to exercise every day doesn't hold up on the French Riviera Body Program, because this program doesn't require lots of time. The old half-hour-or-nothing drill and the "more is better" philosophy aren't very French Riviera, where a little of a good thing is considered better than nothing at all or a lot of nothing; quality is more important than quantity.

Maybe you're setting your daily goals too high. The French Riviera Body isn't one particular feeling or look. It's a combination of image, physicality, and mental attitude, all at their best. Remember, too, you don't have to exercise for the same amount of time each day.

If you're still shaking your head and sighing, "No, I just don't have the time, I really don't," then construct your own chart of a typical day's activities. See if you are spending too much time doing any one thing. Try taking a minute, just one minute, of the time you spend doing errands or housework, making telephone calls, writing letters, attending meetings, and shopping. If you try, I'm sure you'll be able to come up with at least five extra minutes every day.

Q. *Is there a point at which you reach a plateau and you can't progress anymore?*
A. Exercising becomes easier. For example, you feel certain stretches less intensely and you can exercise for longer periods of time before you feel mildly fatigued, but you never stop progressing. And you never reach a plateau while you're on this program. There's always room for improvement in how you do the exercises and how true you are to yourself about following this program exactly as described. The French Riviera Body always has something new to aim for and achieve.

You will notice your progress daily; it will be most evident each time you start the weekly cycle of exercising. But while you discover that what may have been difficult or nearly impossible to accomplish the week(s) before is becoming more attainable and even surpassable, you will also realize how much more there is to strive for.

Q. *Some sessions seem harder to me than others. Are they?*
A. No, they're all of equal substance, although some sessions will seem more difficult to different people. How you perceive what is difficult or easy depends on what your own developed or inherited weaknesses and strengths are. For you, bending forward might be quite a strenuous movement, and sit-ups so easy you could do them in your sleep. For someone else, it could be the reverse.

Q. *It never fails. The minute I start exercising, my children want something to eat, the phone rings, the doorbell chimes. Something always seems to get in the way or interrupt me when I'm exercising or just about to start. Do these interruptions reduce the effectiveness of the program?*
A. It's minimal, but interruptions do reduce some of the effectiveness of this program, since they prevent you from exercising in the sustained manner that leads to a stronger cardiovascular system and increased stamina, strength, speed, coordination, fluidity of movement, and grace. And they divert your attention from the program and your body, causing you to lose momentum, motivation, time, and your chance to adhere to your exercise schedule. Examine the chart. Revise your schedule if at all possible to avoid constant interruptions.

Q. *I have a real problem with my waist and stomach. They're extra flabby. What should I do? Do you think they'll ever be firm and trim?*

A. They'll definitely firm up and trim down if you follow this program where every exercise utilizes and benefits those areas in varying degrees.

Keep in mind that the way in which you exercise as well as the way in which you apply what you learn from this program in your everyday life affects your appearance, health, sense of well-being, the speed with which you achieve the French Riviera Body, and, since you asked, how trim and firm your waist and stomach do become. So as you exercise—and even when you're not exercising—be sure always to pull your abdominal muscles in toward your back and up toward your ribs. Lift your weight up off your hips; feel that space between your hips and ribs smooth out, firm up, and trim down. That's the secret to attaining and then maintaining a flat stomach and a trim waistline.

Q. *On the St. Tropez Body Plan, why do we have to do the wind-ups and the wind-down with each day's session? Why don't we just do the wind-ups before the first day's session and the wind-down after the second day's session?*
A. The wind-up and wind-down exercises are beneficial to you; they improve the quality with which you start, repeat, or finish the sessions. And, on the French Riviera Body Program, the quality of the exercises (and exercising) and attaining the best results go hand in hand.

Q. *When I think of exercise, I think of how it will make me look: Will it make me thinner, etc.? You talk so much about flexibility, coordination, strength, and stamina. What do they have to do with looking good?*
A. Looking good is not a body that's weak, sluggish, stiff, and tired. What's the beauty in looking good if you can't bend and stretch or don't have the strength or endurance to work, play, love, live, and be with people?

Looking good is looking, feeling, and being alive. It's much more than a thin body. (Skeletons are thin; a lot of good it does them.) In fact, the French Riviera Body can have a few more pounds on it. A body being exercised on the French Riviera Body Program redistributes its fat and shapes up its muscles in such a no-nonsense way that a few extra pounds are not unsightly. Besides, you're not a mannequin. Thin and trim is a waste of time—and it's not attractive—if there's no vitality, confidence, or agility attached to it.

Much more than a trim waistline, flat stomach, sleek hips, firm arms, tight derrière, the French Riviera Body Program also gives you increased agility and stamina and a look and feeling of confidence. On this program you don't just change flabbiness and fatness to firmness and trimness, you change your perspective and your body for the better. You give your life a new sense of purpose and meaning. You create a body that doesn't just look great but also moves well, stands beautifully, sits gracefully, and has the stamina and will to do much more than exercise.

By following this program exactly as described, you can improve the quality of your life forever. For instance, coordination, which is vital to productivity, is enhanced through each exercise. Scientific studies have shown that as the human body ages, the central nervous system deteriorates; therefore, one's central nervous system needs to be kept active and challenged throughout one's life in order to preserve its abilities and fortify its strengths.

Q. *What kind of music do you suggest we use?*
A. Any music you like. Sometimes music with a strong rhythm gives you a pace to follow. I use anything from classical to jazz to rock music.

Q. *Can I follow the French Riviera Body Program one day or a few days a week and the St. Tropez Body Plan on the other days?*
A. Yes. Let common sense, your chart, and your body guide you.

Q. *I used to be in shape; then I stopped exercising because I changed jobs, couldn't get to classes, got married and moved out of my apartment. How long will it take me to get back in shape on the French Riviera Body Program?*
A. It all depends on the kind of shape you were in before you stopped exercising, how long ago you stopped exercising, how old you are, what your goals are, how much time you intend to exercise every day, and so forth. Of course, it also depends on the condition you're in now and how long you've been in that condition.

I can't tell you exactly how long it will take you to get back into shape. But you can use my "optimum, excellent, and very good" guidelines to give you an approximation.

116

Q. *Is it dangerous to skip a day of exercises? Sometimes everything hurts and I'm so stiff, I just don't feel like doing it.*

A. The danger lies in the fact that you will break up your routine and lose the habit of following this program daily on a regular basis.

Once you start skipping days and following this program sporadically—when you feel like it, when you're in the mood for it—you'll find it harder to do the exercises, get any results, and stay on this program. With each passing day, you'll allow yourself to lose some strength, stamina, and flexibility.

Q. *Is it possible to use any of your exercises as spot reducers?*

A. The French Riviera Body Program is a complete exercise regimen for the total you. Each exercise has been integrated into the program with this goal in mind. Therefore, I don't recommend trying to pick and choose among the exercises for panaceas to particular complaints. You are more likely, as I've explained earlier, to lose interest in the program when you abandon the careful structure than you are to solve your specific problem.

117

	Dates	Time	Where
MONDAY			
TUESDAY			
WEDNESDAY			
THURSDAY			
FRIDAY			
SATURDAY			
SUNDAY			

With Whom   *Comments*